MICROPENIS:

The Long and Short of It

David Brian

ISBN: 1500610038
ISBN 13: 9781500610036

Library of Congress Control Number: 2014913149
CreateSpace Independent Publishing Platform
North Charleston, South Carolina

Contents

Micropenis and the Damage Done

My self-published book *Penoplasty: A True Story* was my first attempt at writing a book. Although there were some errors that crept in, I put my heart and soul into it. It was what it said on the tin—it was a true story. Most of the book was about my struggle living with a micropenis, which I called my one-inch stump. Hopefully my first book explained that it wasn't exactly a barrel of laughs. My very first dance with a girl wasn't until I was 25 and that was with a lesbian- her girlfriend was standing there peeing herself with laughter!

That said, my advisor—if I can call her that—Sally Morgan, suggested that I should add some humorous parts to lighten the load of telling people what a terrible existence it is to have such a tiny manhood. Even in the darkest of moments, there can be light, and you can find the relief of humour if you look deeply enough. So I hope that some lighter moments appeared through the darker, more painful parts of the book.

Sally is a true artist with words, which is probably why she's a freelance journalist. Besides wanting a much bigger penis, I only wish I could express myself like Sally. Life's so unfair, but I mustn't let that take me into one of my depressive moments. I will say that Sally has not helped me in writing this book and that she has not recommended this book in any way. She has, however, written a few words about her interview with me back in 2002.

When I was trying to find a British book publisher who would be prepared to promote my story, most wouldn't touch it with a bargepole. Some replied to my letter and attached synopsis and gave me some optimism by saying something like, 'There's potential for an interesting story, but unfortunately it's not one we feel our company could promote.' One book company in Brighton, England, asked me to send the full draft of my book, which gave me some real optimism. They eventually replied saying they liked my story, although they thought my third chapter ('TV Highlights') was too lengthy, and they could publish my book. However, the sting in the tail was that I would have to pay them £8,500 for their troubles! You will not be surprised to know I refused their generous offer. I'm certainly not Tony Parsons, English journalist and writer, who could cash in his pension fund to write a book with a well-known publishing company. I'm not in the same league financially as the former New Musical Express (NME) gunslinger. I could only get my book self-published.

Although I've been told by certain persons not to mention that terrible word called money (or even filthy lucre) in my book, I want to give you a true but strange example that really occurred. After my article appeared in the *Daily Mirror*'s *M Magazine* in 2002, a gentleman from the press approached the Belvedere Clinic in South East London, where I had my operations. He contacted me and wanted to make an offer—not to me personally, but to my wife, Shirley. After I had handed the telephone to my wife, he explained that a women's magazine was prepared to offer her £1,000 to tell her story about having a husband who had undergone penis-enlargement surgery. The really strange thing was the magazine wanted a couple of photographs to be included in the article—but the photographs they wanted happened to be of my wife when she was around ten years of age! I found that very odd, to put it mildly.

Micropenis and the Damage Done

Concerning the financial offer, I feel duty-bound to say it was twice as much as I was paid for appearing on television. It just didn't make sense to me at all.

One thing I should explain is that I'm still very envious of the men (all four were black guys) who were mentioned on page 107 of my first book. The TV programme was on channel four under the title *The Biggest Penis in the World*, and it explained that all you had to do was Google bigcocks.com to see magnificently endowed men having sex with extremely attractive women who, as it happened, were all white. I've never looked at that website again (or any other like it) because it crushes your confidence, and I can imagine that even an average man would feel incredibly inferior compared to those sexual supermen. Having said all this, I'm still much more confident after having my operations. Due to my procedures, I might still lag behind the average, but at least I have had my size increased a great deal with the combination of the lengthening procedure and by using the penis stretcher. I'm so glad I had it done.

A few years ago, while researching on the Internet, I discovered that my first interview in August 2002 with Sally Morgan, which originally appeared in the now defunct *Daily Mirror Magazine*, could be seen in its entirety on the 'free library', which is obviously free of charge. My photo doesn't appear with the article, as it did in the magazine, but the full interview is there for all to see. I made Sally aware of this, and we both knew that (sorry to mention money again) we would not be paid any more money for our troubles.

All you have to do to read the article on your computer is to search for any of the following: 'David Turney Embarrassed', 'Sally Morgan Size Matters', 'Sally Morgan Daily Mirror Embarrassed', 'David Turney Size Matters', and 'Size Matters Embarrassed'. These are all variations that will let you read the article in full even though it appeared twelve years ago.

MICROPENIS: The Long and Short of It

For the record, readers of my first book will know that the mere mention of Margi Clarke sends a shiver down my spine. Sally Morgan informed me years ago that she once interviewed Margi about her boudoir, and Sally said she could understand why a bloke like me would be terrified of meeting Margi. For the interview young Margi was dressed to kill, with a pelmet-length dress and high-heeled mules. I'm so glad Sally was the one who interviewed her rather than me!

Regarding this book, I hope it is informative, accurate, and truthful. Despite the newspaper, magazine, radio, and television coverage of penis size and penoplasty (phalloplasty) procedures over the last twenty years, it's still a taboo subject. Trying to break down the taboo is incredibly difficult, and it isn't helped by the dreadful clichés spouted by so-called 'experts', agony aunts and uncles, doctors, and Uncle Tom Cobley and all—the mantra being, of course, 'size doesn't matter; it's what you do with it that counts.' Yeah, and the moon's made out of cheese. If you're a man unfortunate enough to possess a penis smaller than that of a five-year-old boy, it doesn't take a consultant urologist to tell you there's a major problem. Or as we would say these days, it's a problem—big time! The only thing that's big is the problem. I have to say I have seen female to male before and after photographs on You Tube and nearly every penis on show after surgery is big to very big. It's obvious that the women who physically want to be men want a big penis.

Within these pages I've named surgeons who can help men who suffer from micropenis. As I've said before, it isn't compulsory, because if a man is happy with what he's got, so be it. However, if a man is so depressed and worried about having a micropenis, I would like to think he will see where he can go for help.

Since my first operation, I've had dealings with journalists who vary from excellent, like Sally Morgan, to awful—the names will not be mentioned to protect the guilty. I've been interviewed by wonderful television producers, such as the producer of *Drastic Plastic*, to another producer who only wanted every person to adhere to his views on penis size and penis-enhancement surgery. I've often heard that men who come up short in the trouser stakes try to make up with it in other ways, such as bossing people around or thinking their magnetic personality will make them a 'babe magnet'. Pathetic little men like that are so convinced that their fantastic wit and wonderful aura will make their tiny penis something women will not be concerned about. Dream on, you crazy, far-out man!

Mind you, I have to be honest and state that I believe that most poorly endowed men suffer a million times over when it comes to their tiny manhoods. Although most of the stuff on the Internet that can be called 'adult entertainment', or just plain blue or porn movies, worships at the feet of those enormously endowed men, there is another extreme. There seems to be a small niche (pardon the pun) where men with tiny penises are shown with attractive women (mostly fully dressed) who openly mock their miniscule male organs. I'm no expert, but of the few 'films' I've seen of this material, it appears that most of the men's faces are hidden from view. There appears to be some men who do have their faces on camera as well as their tiny organs, but most only have the bottom half of their bodies shown. Perhaps the few men who show their faces as well as their penises are paid extra money for their bravery. It does seem that a large percentage of these men are obese, and the majority cannot even see their own penises when they lay down naked on a bed.

Concerning these films, some people may just see this as a 'jokey' way of laughing at these men, but I find it distasteful in the extreme. The men's penises are often measured, proving that these unfortunates are genuinely owners of micropenises—most only having two or two-and-a-half-inch erect penises. In one or two films the woman indicates how small the man is by measuring the penis with their little finger. Invariably, this is followed by the woman masturbating the man until he ejaculates. The few clips I've seen show the poor man only ejaculating about two spurts of semen. Talk about ridiculing the poor guy. Maybe this is to make up for tons of blue or porn movies where women have appalling things done to them. I've never seen that stuff, and I never will, thank goodness. Nevertheless, it makes me wince when I see these poor men being laughed at. If you want to see these poor blokes, just enter 'tinydicks.com'—have a good laugh, if that's your thing.

Regarding my penoplasty procedures, I will put on record that I paid for every single procedure. I didn't attempt to have my operation on the NHS here in Britain, so no one can accuse me of getting the taxpayers to finance my operations. Most people would be up in arms if the operation came from the NHS coffers. At least you can't point your fingers at me!

One aspect that made me feel extremely proud was when a client of Dr Gary Horn—I have called him RP—contacted me via e-mail about using the Andropenis or the JES Extender. He did say he went ahead with his penoplasty procedure after reading my first book. I felt truly honoured when he informed me of that information. I did say I always cross my fingers when recommending the operation to a man who obviously wants the operation but who is worried about anything going wrong.

Another event that made me feel very proud was when Dr David Veale, a consultant psychiatrist in cognitive behaviour therapy at the South London Maudsley NHS Trust, e-mailed me to say he was impressed by my first book. He also put on record that he thought I was brave to actually write a book about such a sensitive issue.

I've experienced being interviewed for radio as well, which was interesting to say the least. My interview for Radio Scotland lasted about ten minutes and, as far as I'm aware, went without a hitch. The interview before (or possibly after) my interview dealt with a guy who drank his own urine! Apparently it helped his immune system and was beneficial in other ways. Perhaps having your (tiny) penis surgically enlarged isn't so strange after all.

Hopefully you will enjoy reading my book or, at least, find it informative.

A Few Lines from Anna Camilleri

During my active involvement with cosmetic surgery hospitals over the past twelve years and while running my own clinic, I witnessed a massive increase in the popularity of penoplasty procedures. Men from all backgrounds, from the unemployed to barristers, lawyers, and politicians have undergone this procedure so that they can feel better about themselves, increase their confidence, perform better, improve their sexual lives, and give more satisfaction to their partners. Penoplasty also became popular even with guys from the competitive porn industry where, as they say, they are paid by the inch.

Working closely with a surgeon who specialises in penoplasty, I had the opportunity to coach and look after almost two thousand male patients on their journeys to a permanent confidence boost. Although it is a very private and confidential matter to some, there are plenty of guys who admit openly they would like to thicken their penises—not only because it would give them a more attractive, manly look, and undoubtedly increase confidence, but also because it will make for a better sexual experience for them and their partners.

It is no secret that women are attracted to men who project confidence. Nothing can boost manly confidence like exercise and proper grooming and dressing, as well as setting goals and meeting them and learning new skills (outside and inside the bedroom). And when the clothing is taken off and the lights are still on, size is what counts! (For more information on improving male confidence look out for my new book *What Men Want & What Women Want*.)

For all those guys who still walk sadly with their heads down, I am pleased to share the good news! Yes, there are a few temporary nonsurgical ways to thicken your penis; however, they're just temporary. These solutions include pumps, pills, and patches to increase your blood flow, which gives you a thicker appearance. The sad news is that no matter which one of these you choose, you will only get results while you are using them. Once you stop, you are back to square one.

The only permanent method that can give a truly satisfying result for enhancement is penile enlargement surgery, combined with devices (penile stretchers). Using these two methods will give you a thicker, longer penis permanently, providing you follow the postoperative regime and light maintenance programme.

If you have done your research and chosen an experienced surgeon who regularly performs this kind of operation, he (or she) will have given you a set of instructions regarding postoperative care. These instructions are highly important as they refer to the recovery period and must be followed accordingly.

Small Operative Tips:

Once you are back at home after your discharge from the hospital or clinic, rest and do not overexert yourself. If you have booked time off work before your surgery, then make best use of this time and relax. Give yourself time to heal. It is important to massage your penis on a daily basis using Vaseline, which helps to prevent lumps from forming on the surface, and keep the area clean. Do not go swimming or participate in any sports until four to six weeks after surgery.

Many patients ask me how soon they can go to the gym. I normally smile at that question, as I can sense that what they really want to know is how soon they can have sex. Well, if the gym is really your primary concern, then please avoid heavy lifting or any other strenuous activity for a month after surgery. As for any sexual activity, you have to be a bit more patient. It's normally recommended you wait for six weeks before resuming sexual relations.

It is also important to understand that penile surgery will not give overnight results, as it can take from three to six months before you see the full benefits of the surgery.

A Few Lines from Me

I first met Anna Camilleri in 2003 at the Belvedere Clinic, when I had my first consultation with Dr Gary Horn.

What struck me was her friendliness and how she could put me at ease at the time of our first meeting. At that time Anna had already done a procedure together with Dr Horn, which meant she could let me know about his all-round skills as a surgeon.

I found this very reassuring, particularly when I realised I had seen him on a TV documentary performing penile enlargement surgery.

In the end it all worked out wonderfully well, so I was a very happy man.

A Few Lines from Mrs David Brian

Some cosmetic surgery is probably not really required. When David appeared on channel five's *Drastic Plastic*, the black man who had penis enlargement surgery had been confirmed as already having an eight-inch-long penis when erect. He didn't need the operation and had it simply for aggrandisement. David was originally confirmed as having a micropenis and was therefore an ideal candidate for penoplasty. He is so glad to have undergone penile enlargement surgery, and he is extremely happy with the results. I'm also happy—if David's happy, I'm happy.

A Few Lines from Sally Morgan

'Does size matter?' That all depends on the man—and the woman. But it mattered so much to David Brian that he resorted to surgery to enhance what he perceived to be his diminutive masculinity. It had more than the obvious effect on his person, for not only did penoplasty increase the size of his appendage, it also pumped up his self-esteem.

When I first met David in 2002—to interview him for the *Daily Mirror*'s former supplement, *M Magazine*—what struck me most was his courage in confiding in me, a total stranger, about the most intimate part of his anatomy and the misery it had caused. I use the word 'confide', because in fact he knew that thousands of readers would soon know in detail the deepest, darkest humiliation that had haunted him since childhood.

It was a great compliment that he trusted me enough to tell his story to the world through me, and he did so in the hope that it would help other men labouring under the same predicament.

Yet David's passion and bravery doesn't end here. He plucked up the nerve to write a book, *Penoplasty: A True Story*, about how he overcame his ordeal, and through his witty anecdotes and self-effacing humour he raised more than a smile. He also raised hope. Now he has turned to the power of the pen yet again with his second literary offering. So does size matter now? One thing is certain: David has more balls than most!

A Few Lines from a YouGov Survey

A recent YouGov survey's first question was who they would vote for if a General Election took place tomorrow. However, the very last question of the survey (which was on an unrelated subject) asked the question, 'Is penis size important?'

One female respondent replied without hesitation, 'Yes, it is important.' And then she explained that many women are 'brainwashed' to the extent that they feel compelled to pretend that it does not matter.

She added, 'It was certainly a surprise that the question was asked, but, on reflection, maybe the pollster could have been a bit braver and asked a few more questions about this little-debated topic: Would you stay with a guy with a small penis? Should a man with a micropenis be able to have penis-enlargement surgery on the NHS?'

As a man who once possessed a micropenis before I had my operations, I think these questions are important ones that should be addressed. The woman who asked the questions volunteered her own answers. If she met a guy who she really liked, one who was caring and compassionate, one who had a wonderful personality, and one who was very good looking, what would she think if he had one major problem—a tiny penis? She said it was a very difficult question to answer because she wouldn't want to hurt the guy's feelings. But she would have to ask herself one question, would having a very disappointing sex life for the whole of their relationship override all the good points? If she couldn't even feel his penis inside her and he also came in a matter of a couple of seconds, could she live with him? Perhaps not, but she would certainly not say anything nasty to him and would let him down gently. The woman did admit that if another man she met had all the attributes of the first guy but was also well hung and was very satisfying in bed, she would have no hesitation in going out with him.

Regarding the second question, on balance, if the poor man had a genuine micropenis and could not make love to the extent that he was unable to enter her properly and could not even urinate in the normal way, she would agree that he should be able to have penis enlargement surgery on the NHS.

A Few Lines From the Internet—A Lady's Honest Thoughts on Penis Size

'Women, be proud of your preferences', said the subtitle of an in-depth questionnaire regarding women and their preferences when it comes to penis size.

The woman who was organising and collating the information for this website said, 'There were many intelligent replies but also a significant number of replies that followed a troublesome trend. Women who have a preference for the size of their partner's penis size are treated like sluts. If you like big dicks, it means you are a dirty whore who has been stretched out by all the sex you've had. This attitude is just terrible and offensive. The same guys who spend time looking at porn of beautiful, thin women with large breasts are the same guys who will criticise their partner if she hints that she might find larger penises arousing.'

One woman replied to the questionnaire as follows, 'I'm the type who enjoys a little pain with the pleasure, and there's honestly nothing that gets me going more than having someone with a long, thick penis filling me up. That sense of being "full" is something I don't feel with someone smaller.'

Another woman has her say. 'I prefer around six to seven inches, with average girth. Smaller means it just doesn't feel as good, and as a woman who primarily comes from PIV [penis in vagina] sex, it really makes a big difference to me. His tongue rarely does it for me; it has to be dick. I have no issue with being honest about that; it's not putting smaller guys down by me saying the size I prefer.'

A Few Lines from *Psychology Today* on the Internet—Does Penis Size Matter?

'Size does matter. I'm a woman and agree completely with the observations of the other women who have posted here.'

A woman named Annie is very specific and replies as follows, 'Big cocks are much more satisfying than smaller ones. I like at least seven to eight inches and big in girth to fill me up.'

Mary Sojourner states, 'Most of the straight women I've known in years of teaching and leading women's groups have said that when they get honest about intercourse, size matters for their satisfaction. Yes, the clitoris is a prime player in orgasm, but being able to feel your lover's penis "filling" them is another plus in the deal.'

'Mary is correct; I have not met a woman who has said penis size wasn't important when specifically asked about pleasurable sexual intercourse. As a woman it is very important, absolutely no question. The good news is a man doesn't have to be huge, but a three to five inch penis won't do much for a woman's feeling of fullness that we enjoy.'

Dr Gary F Horn, Cosmetic Surgeon

I first met Dr Horn on 6th February 2003 for a consultation concerning my wish for a top-up operation-basically I wanted my girth further enhanced. He read my notes in my folder about my previous penoplasty procedures and questioned me about my current health. After this discussion he examined my penis and he noticed a small but noticeable bump which was a collection of fatty tissue that was a result from my earlier procedure with the previous surgeon. Dr Horn said he could take away the lump for me as well as increase my girth.

Towards the end of our conversation I mentioned that his face was familiar and I wondered if he had been on television. He replied he had been on a BBC programme called "Plastic Fantastic".

As my first book will illustrate the next time I saw him was on 18th June 2003 when he performed my penoplasty in front of the Channel 5 cameras for the documentary "Drastic Plastic" which just goes to show these programmes and titles are variations on a theme. After this he operated on me for my last procedure on 20th October 2005 when I had no cameras spying on me.

I can confirm, without fear of contradiction that both procedures went smoothly (pun intended!) and I had so little bruising it wouldn't be an exaggeration to say I couldn't really see any. I was delighted with the results of both procedures. Fat had been taken from my buttocks and the results were better than the procedures where fat had been taken from the insides of my thighs.

Everyone who wants to see Dr Horn's professional background can check his medical experience online. Briefly I can inform you that he trained in main hospitals in Paris and became a consultant plastic surgeon in 2002 and he now specialises in plastic, aesthetic and reconstructive surgery. Dr Horn has extensive knowledge and experience in all cosmetic surgery. In 2003, he designed the first pectoral implant, which is now used worldwide.

I interviewed Dr Horn in March 2014 when he informed me that he performs approximately 60 penoplasty procedures in a year – he has currently performed about 600 of the procedures. Dr Horn speaks fluent French and English.

Please note that the two photographs on page 66 are of a patient who underwent penoplasty in Dr Horn's clinic in London. The patient gave his permission for the photographs to be published in this book.

A few lines from the Telegraph (online) "Long Story"

"More and more men are turning to penis enlargement or penoplasty, as it is officially termed. So what exactly does penoplasty entail? The Telegraph interviewed a man, identified as 'Dan', who had undergone the surgery three ago. The surgery involved making a small incision at the base of the penis, injecting the removed fat (from Dan's back), then closing the incision. The length of a penis can also be increased through surgery that involves making an incision at the base of the penis, then cutting a ligament that allows the penis to hang 2.5 inches longer. Dan told Telegraph reporters that his penis is now 8 inches erect and roughly the thickness of a Coke can. 'Women tell me it's the fattest dick they have ever seen', Dan said."

For the record Dan is a 50-year-old graphic designer and had his operation at the London Centre for Aesthetic Surgery.

My personal thoughts are that as I only had a one inch penis when flaccid before my first operation in 1996, a micropenis in other words, I would have had no hesitation in going to that clinic to have my penis enlarged. Whatever the cost I would've made damn sure I had enough money for THAT procedure. As history will record I eventually went to the Belvedere Clinic in South East London, but from Dan's experience the London Centre for Aesthetic Surgery would seem to be equally first-rate if you want to have your penis enlarged.

A few lines from Julie Burchill – "Unchosen"

"I'm not boasting or nothing when I say I knew NME (New Musical Express) was going to hire me, because I knew I was a lot cleverer than the dopey halfwits who were running the rag. God, I hated the music, though, and having that needy moron Tony Parsons sniffing around me drove me MAD.

I probably shouldn't have made the mistake of letting him shag me the once, mind, but I like to get pissed me and to be honest, I didn't really know he had shagged me because his cock was so small. After that incident, I wanted a proper Jew because they all have huge cocks."

As I'm not a Jew with a huge cock – in fact as you all know I had a tiny penis – perhaps some of my readers of this book will understand why I had the penoplasty operation as soon as I knew where I could have it done in the UK and, of course, when I had sufficient money.

A few lines from the Telegraph (online) about Russian surgeons

"A Russian man born with genitals so small that he was unable to have sex has been given the chance to lead a normal love life after a new penis was 'grown' on his arm during pioneering surgery.

In an 11-hour operation, surgeons in Moscow removed the 28-year-old's undersized penis and stitched it on to his left forearm, where they grafted on additional flesh and tissue taken from his inner arm. The newly enlarged organ, which had grown from less than 2 inches to nearly 7 inches, was reattached to his groin.

It is thought that up to one in 200 men are born with 'micropenis' - the medical term for male genitalia that are less than two inches long when aroused. Many sufferers find intercourse either difficult or impossible, often having acute psychological problems as a result".

A few lines from Dr Harold Reed, surgeon based in Miami, USA

People who purchased my first book, "Penoplasty: A True Story", will know that Dr Reed is based in Miami and that he was the very first surgeon I read about in the UK's Sun newspaper in July 1991 to have performed penis enlargement surgery. I sent him a complimentary copy of this book and I received the following reply via email: "Good afternoon David. Your new book, "Micropenis: The Long and Short of it", has just been received and I must say I am overwhelmed with your engaging, easy to comprehend literary style and details. This book is being given a very visible place in our medical library. With sincere appreciation, Harold M Reed, M.D."

I, of course, replied thanking Dr Reed for his kind words and support. He has performed the penoplasty (phalloplasty) procedure since 1986 and I have no hesitation in recommending him to any men who want their penis enlarged.

A few lines from Dr Roberto Viel, London Centre for Aesthetic Surgery

"I very much appreciate you sending me your book   -   I found it extremely interesting. I would be happy to mention your book to my patients and have ordered some already to give them in my clinic. Kind regards, Dr Roberto Viel".

It should be noted that Dr Viel has performed penoplasty procedures in his London clinic since 1991. He is vastly experienced in this particular procedure and I can only repeat that I think his excellent results speak for themselves. He is a surgeon who I would give my full recommendation to if you are considering having penoplasty.

A few more lines from Sally Morgan, freelance journalist

I received this email from Sally Morgan on 1st February 2015, "Dear David, Thank you so much for your new book! (It's) so well written and in a lovely, witty, readable style. A big thanks too, for the complimentary comments you made about me – I'm touched! Hope all is well with you and yours. Best wishes Sally M".

From my point of view I cannot believe there's a more talented writer than Sally. She's been a journalist for 25 years or more and during that time she has interviewed many very famous people – including Margi Clarke who would frighten the life out of me if I ever met her in person. On the other hand Sally has also written articles about ordinary people who have interesting, or sometimes extraordinary stories to tell. As far as I'm concerned if a newspaper, magazine or journal wants a story written to the highest standard they need not look any further than Sally.

A few lines from Vanessa Engle – about her documentary concerning Harley Street, London on BBC2 April 2015

"The people who take part in documentaries - or at least in my documentaries – are very altruistic. I don't think any of them are doing it because they want to be on television. If they were, I wouldn't include them. I think they want to take part because they are going through something difficult and they want to share that experience, so that other people have a better understanding. People's own lives are very precious to them and they want to explain".

CHAPTER ONE

Testimonials

As my previous book, *Penoplasty: A True Story,* stated, I had my first peno-plasty operation on August 13, 1996. This was my most major operation because the surgeon both lengthened and thickened my penis. It was also one of the most important events in my life, because I suffered from what is called micropenis.

The only things in my life more important have been

1) the day my beloved mother died,

2) witnessing the birth of my beautiful daughter, and

3) marrying my wife on my wedding day.

Nothing else comes close—although I must say that appearing on UK national television (two different documentaries on channel five and BBC3) and having my story told in a number of magazine articles certainly caused my heart to beat much faster. Being recognised by peo-ple for no other reason than having my penis enlarged is unbelievably unnerving. What's worse is being recognised by people who *do* know me. Please take my word for it. Brave or mad? I'll leave it up to you, dear reader, to make up your own mind.

To all the male readers of this book I would ask you these questions: Would you be interviewed on mainstream television, discussing how your penile enlargement operation had gone? Not only that, would you be willing to stand completely naked in front of the cameras? Would you allow the cameras to show your penoplasty operation, which was making your penis thicker?

Only you can answer these questions. The female producer of the channel five documentary (or cockumentary, as some comedians have called it) said I was definitely 'brave'. Her opinion was that many men have this procedure, but very few would be honest and brave enough to discuss their penis enlargement surgery in front of the cameras.

Forgetting for a moment interviews with print and visual media, the facts are these. I was in the bottom 3 percent of men when it came to the size of my manhood, and it hurt psychologically like you just wouldn't believe. You have to experience it to understand the overwhelming sense of inadequacy.

The problem is that the other 97 percent of men would not fully understand how a man like me would feel. Would I really understand how it would feel to live on the streets, sleeping in a shop doorway at night? I could try, but the odds are that I just wouldn't be able to comprehend the degradation of it all.

Regarding the television documentary *Drastic Plastic*, which I appeared on, I can state quite categorically that the TV producer was absolutely trustworthy and totally professional in everything she did concerning my story in her programme.

I still blush when I think about the section of the documentary when my penoplasty procedure was shown for the whole of Britain to see. The producer was there, witnessing it *all* as she stood in the operating theatre at the Belvedere Private Clinic in South East London. And I'll add that it certainly made my face red as a beetroot thinking about the million-plus people who watched the first airing of the programme.

The producer totally understood my embarrassment, and the biggest compliment I can give her is that I felt I could trust her completely. She was a real sweetie, to quote a phrase, and I'm sure her career will get ever more impressive as time goes on.

Testimonials

She was quite obviously a very experienced and extremely talented producer and director who has been good enough to communicate with me several times since the programme was shown. Why aren't there more human beings like her?

On the other hand the producer of the TV programme on BBC3, who himself had a small penis (but not as small as mine), was nowhere near as pleasant and certainly wasn't as trustworthy as the female producer. The man, who BBC3 had allowed to produce his own documentary/cockumentary about penis size, had his own agenda and then some. The hour-long interview I had with him in no way reflected the true nature of our discussion. I felt cheated. I still do.

The only clip shown of me that was truly representative of my feelings was the opening scene when I announced, 'It's not much fun having a small one. I don't care what anyone tells me.' The rest of my interview, edited down to two minutes, was the producer's attempt to pretend I wasn't happy with the result of my five operations. That simply wasn't the case, and it just goes to show that not every TV producer will tell the whole truth and nothing but the truth.

I remember David Bowie on the BBC documentary *Cracked Actor,* saying in an exaggerated cockney accent, 'Honest, guv (governor), I wasn't even there.' The trouble with me was that I was there—on a TV screen near you with over one million people watching. It may now be history, but it's history I will *never* forget.

As for magazine articles, the standout journalist by a country mile was Sally Morgan. Sally's very intelligent and can write wonderfully well. She also possesses the great empathy to understand a person's problems, both physical and emotional.

My first interview with her, which took place in my house, was extremely sensitive and incredibly personal. Like the female TV producer, Sally has this wonderful knack of dealing with ordinary people who have, shall we say, extraordinary stories to tell.

MICROPENIS: The Long and Short of It

After the first article appeared in print, we went through a difficult time, because my wife wasn't sure that I had done the right thing in going through with the interview. Over time she has accepted that it was something I wanted to do—even if I wasn't exactly 100 percent confident myself at the time.

Other journalists I have had experience with, although they were not bad (except one), were certainly not in the same class as Sally. How I envy Sally's ability to write factual stories. She has the ability to use the right words, never too many and never too few. To my mind this is an art form and Sally is an artist with words.

After my first operation in 1996, I was asked by the then patient coordinator of the clinic, Glyn Drewe, if I was prepared to write a testimonial. She knew I was very happy with the results of my operation. I felt very honoured to undertake what is, after all, an important task. I knew I had to tell the truth, and to choose my words carefully.

I asked myself these following questions: Was I happy with the increase in my penis size? Absolutely! was the enthusiastic answer. Would I recommend the surgeon and the clinic? Yes I would, with no hesitation. Was I nervous about having the operation? I was petrified, and that is the honest answer—but I wanted it so much. Was it painful? Yes, to an extent but not too painful. I have a low threshold for pain and if I could handle the discomfort anyone could.

The other important thing was that I followed the advice of the surgeon and nursing staff to the letter. I took my medication and painkillers as prescribed. I bathed in a prescribed solution (the surgeon said it helped the healing process) for the duration of my recovery.

Finally, would I recommend the operation to other men? Yes, I would, as long as the man wanted it for himself. If his wife, girlfriend, or partner also wanted him to have the operation, then I would tell him to go ahead. If you're absolutely sure you want or need the enlargement operation, go for it, because if you don't, you might regret it for rest of your life. But on the other hand, if you have too many doubts don't do it. You'll know yourself if it's for you.

I will write a few paragraphs that all men wishing to have this operation should take note of. Do not have unrealistic expectations about the extra size you will gain by having only *one* operation.

In May 2013 I had a conversation with Anna Camilleri, previously of the Belvedere Clinic in South East London, now running the Mayfair Clinic at 100 Harley Street in London. The surgeon performing penoplasty operations and other procedures at the clinic is Dr Gary Horn.

Anna has worked with Dr Horn since April 2002. She has seen many clients come through the doors of various clinics. She has now arrived at the conclusion that whilst men should properly vet a clinic and surgeon, the clinic and surgeon should, when necessary, vet one or two of the clients. Perception, as they say, is everything.

Anna described how an unnamed client, couldn't wait to have his penis enlarged surgically, but didn't have the good sense to follow the precise instructions of the surgeon. The man barely left it forty-eight hours after having surgery before phoning Anna explaining that he was worried because he still had some bruising and swelling on his penis!

No matter how much Anna tried to reassure him, he cried like a baby. If only the man had understood the details of the procedure itself and the postop aftercare that had been explained to him by Dr Horn at the time of his consultation.

Another man, who apparently seems to have lost touch with reality, couldn't understand why the healing process was taking longer than a couple of days. He also had totally unrealistic expectations of the sort of increase he was likely to receive.

I don't want to sound as if I'm totally unsympathetic to these two men, but they should have had the *nous* to follow the step-by-step list of instructions given to them before the operation. As with any surgery, a patient should always heed the advice and instructions of the surgeon.

MICROPENIS: The Long and Short of It

Poor Anna had gone away with her children for an extended weekend only to find she was taking calls from these men morning, noon, and night. She did her best to calm them down and encourage them to wait a few weeks for the results of the procedure to become evident and for healing to begin.

These men should have read and understood the FAQ section of the Mayfair clinic's website, found at www.penilesurgerylondon.co.uk.

My first book is advertised on the website, but I must stress that I'm not being paid to advertise the Mayfair clinic. However, I'm not afraid to say I recommend Anna as a specialist in the cosmetic surgery field, and I have no problem in recommending Dr Horn as a penoplasty surgeon.

I will explain my own experiences. After I had my first operation in August 1996, I was given a list of dos and don'ts as well as a prescription for antibiotics and painkillers. As it was my first, and most invasive, operation, I experienced a fair amount of bruising and a small amount of swelling. The pain, as mentioned before, was noticeable, but in all honesty it wasn't too bad. As research has shown, chronic migraine sufferers like me do feel other pains more acutely than others. If I can put up with the discomfort of penoplasty, anyone can.

Regarding size expectations: I was tiny—only one inch when flaccid. After my operation, my size doubled, so that I was two inches when flaccid. This is the *truth* and nothing but the truth. I was *very* happy with the results.

I will explain about the two operations performed on me by Dr Horn in June 2003 and October 2005. Both procedures produced excellent results. He harvested fat from my buttocks, which was excellent for thickening my penis. The fat obtained from my buttocks was of better quality than the fat obtained from my inner thighs. That's a fact, not an opinion.

The two operations Dr Horn performed on me left me with little or no bruising. In fact I was shocked that the bruising could hardly be seen.

Testimonials

When I saw Dr Horn on October 5, 2011 at the Welbeck Hospital, he informed me that *all* the fat obtained in 2003 and 2005 will remain with me for the rest of my life. Since my first operation in 1996 my girth has therefore been *doubled*. That's a statement of fact. I left the clinic that day with a smile on my face.

Unfortunately some men do not listen properly when being told information that's important. What is it with some men? I'm not very intelligent, but even I could understand what the surgeon was telling me—and I could understand when to take my medication.

You also have to be patient. I was clearly told I should wait for about six weeks before having sexual intercourse. I waited eight weeks, as I'd rather be safe than sorry. The way I looked at it, I had waited forty-two years for *that* operation. Another couple of weeks wouldn't hurt.

Going back to my first book, I would refer you to pages 94 and 95, wherein I interviewed Dr Horn and discovered that only five percent of men were disappointed with the results of their penoplasty. Dr Horn could have lied and pretended that 100 percent of men were unbelievably happy with the results. In fact, it would have been exactly that— unbelievable. I'm sure Dr Horn would love to have 100 percent of his patients happy with their penoplasty procedure, but that would be a dream, and only a dream.

My advice to the underendowed men out there is this. If you decide to have the operation, listen carefully to what the surgeon has to say. Take your time and don't get impatient because you want the healing process to speed up. If you've got any questions ask the surgeon or nurse. Take your medication when it is required and rest for as long as it takes. Thus endeth the first lesson.

My first testimonial, written in December 1996 was as follows:
> When my wife and I saw an advertisement in the *Daily Mirror* regarding penile enlargement undertaken at the Belvedere Private Clinic, my wife contacted the clinic for information and literature.

MICROPENIS: The Long and Short of It

After my consultation in April 1996 I eventually had my operation in August 1996. The feelings of elation I had in the recovery room after I pulled up my gown to see my bandaged but obviously enlarged penis was almost impossible to describe.

My wife and I are very happy with the results of the operation. The psychological boost of having a larger penis has been immense—I feel so much more confident as a man.

When my wife checked my increased size with a tape measure, it was worth more than money could buy. Needless to say the operation was worth every penny. My only regret is that I couldn't have had the operation done years ago.

The surgeon, clinic, matron, nursing staff, and all the ladies in the Patient Services office were all first-rate and extremely helpful.

I would recommend the operation to any underendowed man or to one not confident about his size. I remember someone saying, 'Remember, the tape measure and ruler doesn't lie.'

I have always worried about my tiny penis. From my schooldays to the present day, my condition is known as 'micropenis'. My feelings of inadequacy have been made worse when seeing, reading, or hearing about well endowed men—stories about well-hung males being so much more prevalent nowadays.

The zoologist and anthropologist Desmond Morris said, 'A curious myth perpetuated by modern sex manuals is that human penis size is unimportant. This appears to be a sop to protect the egos of those males likely to need to read such books. The simple fact is that a larger penis is physically more stimulating to the human female, although it goes without saying that a much-loved male with a small penis will be more arousing then a little-loved male with a large one. However, given equal emotional attachment, the bigger penis will always win.'

I'm glad I've had the operation.

Testimonials

My second testimonial, written in January 2013, was as follows:

I had my first penoplasty procedure (both lengthening and thickening) at a clinic in South East London on August 13, 1996. I was very satisfied with the results performed by the then-resident surgeon.

However, on June 18, 2003 I had a 'top-up' performed by a new surgeon, namely Dr Gary Horn. I could hardly forget the day, as my story and operation were filmed by cameras for a documentary on channel five.

Naturally I was very nervous, particularly with a film crew following me around, but Dr Horn put me very much at ease. After the operation I came round to discover the results were first rate. Dr Horn had taken fat from one of my buttocks to further increase my girth and this method proved to be very successful.

I should also mention Anna Camilleri, who was the then Patient Coordinator at the clinic. She was extremely helpful and pleasant to talk to. She explained everything in clear, concise language, and I really recommend her as a consultant.

Finally, I will say that I had one last 'top-up' performed by Dr Horn in October 2005, which further increased my girth. I saw Dr Horn in October 2011, when I told him I had retained all the fat he had harvested in the two procedures he had performed. The best news from Dr Horn was that I would retain *all* the fat for the rest of my life. That was wonderful news.

I should say there's no such thing as an operation without any risks—there's no such thing as a 100 percent completely safe operation. What you can do, though, is use a surgeon with an excellent track record and one who has a detailed consultation about the procedure. Where possible have a word with previous patients who have had experience of the surgeon.

I can speak from personal experience and say I remain extremely grateful that Dr Horn performed both my procedures.

MICROPENIS: The Long and Short of It

I have written a book about my experiences entitled *Penoplasty: A True Story,* and I truly think it's an honest account of how my operations, performed by Dr Horn, have given me extra confidence.

There are some slight differences in the two testimonials but then again, seventeen years, give or take, is quite a long time between the times when I took stock of my perceptions. The common thread between the two testimonials is that I remain very happy with the results of my five operations. The last two operations, with previous experience behind me, gave me far less physical concerns than the first three procedures. As you get older some things become easier.

I do feel sorry for the two men who were clearly frightened out of their minds about the results of their operations. However, they must count to ten, or a hundred if need be, before making a judgement on their respective operations. Rome wasn't built in a day, and the men should wait a reasonable time (six weeks say) to let their penises heal properly. Then they should wait long enough before judging the increase in length and girth that they have gained—leave that for between two and three months. Further gains to their length will be made when they use the penis stretcher. Yes folks, it really works. Details will follow later in this book.

CHAPTER TWO

Television History Made

On July 11, 2012, UK daytime-television history was made when 'Danny' was interviewed about his penoplasty operation.

This took place on ITV's programme *This Morning*, when Philip Schofield and Holly Willoughby interviewed a man called 'Danny'—although that was not his real name—about his penoplasty operation. He decided to remain anonymous and kept his back to the camera for the whole interview. To help keep his identity a secret, he even wore a wig.

The person that did face the camera, however, was his surgeon, Dr Roberto Viel, who helped the interview process by explaining the procedure for lengthening and thickening of the penis. He informed viewers that he'd been doing this procedure since 1991, and he was currently performing about five operations a week. He informed Philip Schofield that men of all ages and backgrounds had the procedure. From young men to retired old uns and from self-employed builders to professional classes, they all wanted to have it done.

The programme called it, somewhat euphemistically, a 'manhood makeover', but it had no need to be so coy about the subject matter. When presenters Richard and Judy were at the helm of the show in 1992, they interviewed two men who had also undergone penis enlargement surgery. The men had also had their backs to the cameras, so shame has not changed much in twenty years.

What has changed is this. Those two British blokes had to travel to America to have the operation. What else? Well, this time, Danny's before-and-after photographs of his penis were shown on our TV screens and, of course, on the Internet. Some things do change over time.

Before I explain more about the media coverage of this particular piece of TV history, I will state openly that I envied Danny's penis size *before* he had girth enhancement. As for his size after the procedure I really feel I don't have to explain. He's a lucky so-and-so and that's no lie.

But I will maintain that I'm very happy with the results of the procedures I had done. The only pity from my perspective is that Danny had such a head start over me to begin with. Danny certainly didn't suffer from 'micropenis'.

There was a humorous part of the programme. It was noticed by several people, including Ms Willoughby, that Danny's grey-coloured wig and his pink shirt made him look a bit like Philip Schofield! Danny's interview was a prerecorded segment from the previous week so Mr Schofield should have realised that when he introduced the piece a week later a pink shirt was a definite no-no.

Here's some more rib-tickling fun. An online report from the *Daily Mail* reported this part of daytime TV history with the headline, 'A man identified as Danny on This Morning said he was suffering from "penis dysmorphia". He blames women, society and the media for "toxic" attitudes to penis size.' Make of that what you will!

The author of the online piece, Peter Lloyd, wrote, 'Breaking new ground for prewatershed viewing, this nine-minute feature peaked when before-and-after photos flashed up on screen; no doubt to cackles of laughter in the production office and across the country.'

He acknowledged Danny as a 'fellow men's activist' and said he saluted his bravery. Mr Lloyd thought that Danny did not undergo the operation for vanity or in order to outdo his mates in the changing room. Furthermore, he thought Danny did not have penoplasty to correct a medical problem which was blighting his life—Mr Lloyd said it wouldn't have been taken seriously even if he had.

This is my opinion on the programme and the aftermath. I'd not heard this phrase 'penis dysmorphia' before and I don't care for it much personally. As for Danny not trying to out-do his mates in the changing room, how the hell does Mr Lloyd know that? Listen, men are notoriously competitive—particularly in the changing room. Has Mr Lloyd not heard of the condition called 'locker-room syndrome'?

As for people laughing at before-and-after photographs, well, let them laugh. I acknowledge that as well as not being intelligent I'm also not very brave. I did shudder and feel incredibly embarrassed after my body and penis was shown on the channel five documentary *Drastic Plastic*. However, as I get older, I just think if they want to laugh at my small penis that's fine by me. Well, it's not something I will actually enjoy, but I have to accept life's not always fair. Have a good laugh at my expense if you really want to, but I bet you're not perfect.

What is Mr Lloyd going on about? According to Mr Lloyd, this chap Danny has started a new political movement for men. Apparently Mr Lloyd wants men to join as one to combat all those nasty women out there who tease and make fun of men with small penises. Not only that, Mr Lloyd thinks many women make fun of penises *per se*. You women out there are really awful!

Mr Lloyd explained that as a man he has many close female friends and women in his immediate family—women who are often smart, successful and emotionally intelligent—but around 90 percent of whom have offended him at some point by mocking another guy's penis. He then says that he was at a friend's twenty-first birthday party which was festooned with pictures of his friend at various stages of his life. One photo was of Mr Lloyd's friend as a baby being washed in a baby-sized bath. Naturally, as a baby the chap had a very small appendage, which one woman noticed and giggled, 'I see he hasn't changed much, if you know what I mean!'

I would say to Mr Lloyd that women have had to put up with men over the centuries voicing their opinions about women's bodies—this including those they know and those they don't know. Men have said these things aloud for everybody to hear. These men haven't cared tuppence about women's feelings. What about the times when men from the building site wolf-whistle and make stupid comments like, 'Get yer tits out for the lads', when an attractive woman walks past.

As for me, I remember well one comment. I didn't lose my virginity until I was thirty years of age. The young lady, named Debbie, was very attractive and she actually told me she couldn't feel my penis inside her, because it was too small. I felt absolutely devastated upon being told this. But even with this, I would not say anything nasty about her. As an American would probably say, 'It hurts like hell being told that but for heaven's sake she's only telling the *truth*.'

To finish off the fun bit we'll look at the comments made by some women on the *Sun* online. One women observed, 'Holly [Willoughby] couldn't take her eyes off the before-and-after shots and had a funny smirk on her face.'

Another woman said, 'People that say "It is all in how you use it" have small ones. That's all there is to it. I have never met anyone that would *prefer* a small one. It is a natural instinct for a woman to want a big one, the same as when a man wants a woman with a large bosom.'

Quite by chance, at the same time Danny was telling Britain about his 'manhood makeover', the *Sun* ran a story ('Breast of British') about Chantal Marshall, fifty-three years old, who had undergone four breast enlargements to increase her breast size from 34B to 32GG. Not only that, she had four daughters who had also undergone breast-enhancement operations, and they, as a family, posed for the paper in their bikinis. The daughters, ranging in age from twenty-one to thirty, joined their mum in the photo shoot, and they all appeared with happy, smiling faces. Chantal's youngest daughter, who was only fourteen, was already talking about having her breasts enlarged when she reached eighteen years of age.

Now, I do have to say that all the women involved in this story had no hesitation in facing the camera and having their real names, including their surnames, published in the best-selling UK newspaper. Their whole attitude seemed to be, 'What's there to worry about? We wanted our breasts enlarged, and we went ahead and had the operation. So what?'

Many women commenting on Danny's operation couldn't understand why he wouldn't face the camera. Is it that penis size, penis enlargement operations, and everything concerning the male organ is still taboo in the twenty-first century? As far as I'm concerned, the subject of the male organ still causes people to either convulse with laughter or to write snotty letters to the media saying, 'Stop all this nonsense; this is an outrage which offends public morals.'

One other point I should address is the subject of the TV watershed. I had wondered, on seeing the penoplasty segment on *This Morning*, if the television watershed no longer applied. In this regard I e-mailed the female producer of *Drastic Plastic* to find out how a professional from the television industry viewed this subject.

The producer replied as follows, 'I'm not sure I'm the best qualified to comment on [the] watershed really. It's more a compliance issue (I'd go to Compliance at ITV with my programme to get advice about what can be shown and what time). But for what it's worth, the watershed is still very much in effect. Quite often, even when a programme is postwatershed, if there is particularly shocking imagery or language in it I will be given advice to put that element of the programme—a sort of sliding scale, so the later it's shown, the less likely it will be seen by those who shouldn't be watching (minors). However, I suspect in the case of the programme you mention they will have sought editorial justification, as

MICROPENIS: The Long and Short of It

I presume the item dealt with male health so was in the public interest. On these occasions, I believe dispensations can be made as long as they meet a certain criteria and the necessary verbal or on screen warnings are included so that those who chose not to watch (or to allow their children to watch) can turn off or turn over. So I guess that's what happened there. Though I didn't see it (or work on it), so can't say for sure.'

There you have the expert opinion on the matter, although I've a feeling the producer concerned would perhaps deny having expertise! Whatever she thinks, I really do believe she has given me an excellent description of how things work in the television industry when it comes to sensitive issues being shown on our TV screens.

If I've understood her comments correctly, and there are legitimate health (or emotional/psychological) issues, the programme will get clearance to be shown on our screens as long as there is a prior warning of the adult nature of the upcoming clips. By clips I think I mean photographs and/or language. As the producer says, the programme on *This Morning* was considered to be dealing with something in the public interest.

All this leaves me wondering why the subject of the male organ can't be dealt with in a sensible and adult fashion. There have been exceptions to the rule—for example, when my story was being discussed on channel five's *Drastic Plastic* and when Sally Morgan wrote so eloquently about my operations.

It does seem a gender thing, with women's body issues being discussed in a much more adult and sensitive way than when the topic in question covers the male body—particularly when the subject matter is a man's penis.

I've seen the segment from *This Morning* about Danny's operation. When asked by Holly and Philip about his procedure he confirmed he was very happy with the results. As he explained there were no 'foreign' bodies used to thicken his penis. Furthermore there were no 'lumps or bumps' as a result of his operation. He mentioned that there might be some absorption of the fat transferred to enhance his penis. However, Dr Viel has sufficient reserves of Danny's fat in order to enhance the penis size back to the postop dimension without any further cost. Amazingly, he informed Holly that he had sexual intercourse only two weeks after his operation! I waited eight weeks to ensure there were no problems with my healing process. I would opt on the side of caution, but it obviously depends on the individual.

Lastly, Dr Viel informed the viewers that most men kept news of their penoplasty very private. That's something that I've been acutely aware of.

On June 28, 2012, there was an article in the *Sun* about Dr Roberto Viel and the penoplasty operation. The headline was, 'I Didn't Want to Be "Mr Average": Fat From My Love Handles Made Me Big Downstairs'. Reading the article, it all seems similar to *This Morning's* segment about 'Danny'. In the article the man was named Mark Edwards, but at the end of the article there was a note saying, 'Names have been changed'. The article said that Mark Edwards's penis measures six and a half inches long, but he wanted to have a thicker girth, which was exactly what the operation gave him. To quote the article, 'He was thrilled.'

What I liked about the piece is that the resident *Sun* doctor, Dr Carol Cooper, had this to say, 'Some procedures use the patient's own fat, others rely on human tissue banks. Whichever way it is done, it is a major op and can have serious risks. One is infection, either at the site of the op or where the graft was taken. Another possibility is that the graft does not "take", leaving an unsatisfactory result. But, when it works well, the patient is usually very pleased. Only surgeons who are experienced in this type of op should be doing these procedures. In skilled hands, a realistic result would be a 30 percent girth increase, and for lengthening ops, an increase of one to two inches.'

As I was finishing this book, guess what news arrived hot off the press? How is this for a headline: 'Penis Size: Meet The Man Who Had Penoplasty Surgery To Make His Ten-Inch Manhood Even Bigger.' This was the headline on the *Huffington Post* website which explained that one Billy-Tom O'Connor, who already had a Ten-inch penis, underwent penoplasty to have his girth further enhanced so he would end up with 'a monster'.

The story was broadcast on July 1, 2014 on ITV's *This Morning*, with presenters Holly Willoughby and Philip Schofield asking questions of Mr O'Connor and the surgeon, who was none other than Roberto Viel. It was announced that over the last year, demand for the penis-enlargement operation has risen by 40 percent, and Billy-Tom O'Connor happened to be one of those who were demanding it.

The only difference was that Billy-Tom already possessed a penis measuring ten inches in length when erect, although he wanted to have a bigger girth so he could claim to have a monster. To illustrate how big Billy-Tom was after the operation, Philip Schofield 'whacked out a hairspray can to demonstrate the size of Billy-Tom's penis when erect.' Lengthwise it measures ten inches, and its girth now measures seven and a half inches around.

The whole interview is available on the Internet, where you will see that viewers were warned that they would see before-and-after pictures of his member. As it said on the *Huffington Post* website, 'In what was certainly a TV shocker, ITV showed before and after shots of Billy-Tom's flaccid penis before and after surgery at the early time of 11:30 a.m., way before the 9:00 p.m. watershed.'

Unlike 'Danny', who made television history with his back to the camera while wearing a wig, Billy-Tom showed that he had no such worries. He sat facing the camera next to Roberto Viel for the whole interview, and he certainly didn't wear a wig. Billy-Tom said that the money he paid for the operation was certainly money well spent—the best value for money he'd ever had.

When Holly Willoughby asked him, 'Is bigger really better?' he replied with no uncertainty that it was. With the exception of two who, upon seeing his 'monster', turned him down, women were extremely happy to take him on.

All I can say is that if 'Danny's' before and after photos left me feeling envious, then Billy-Tom's 'monster' left me feeling like a man with a micropenis, even though I no longer possess one.

Although Billy-Tom had a dodgy haircut—a mullet style—he oozed confidence, and it is little wonder.

As for the *This Morning* programme, it certainly has a track record for covering eye-catching subjects. There was the first discussion about penoplasty back in 1992 when Richard and Judy interviewed those two who had undergone penis enlargement surgery. As explained, they had their backs to the camera and had to go to America for their enlargement operations.

Then Philip and Holly interviewed the monster of them all—Jonah Falcon—who possesses a thirteen-and-a-half-inch-long erect penis. No wonder he was asked what he had in his pocket when he was at an airport. Talk about a dangerous-looking weapon.

Then we have 'Danny' with his average, made into above-average, penis, after his penoplasty procedure. This has now been followed by Billy-Tom and his ten-inch whopper made into an even bigger 'monster!'

For goodness' sake, all I can ask now is whatever next?

CHAPTER THREE

The History of Penis-Enlargement Surgery and the Clinics that Perform the Operation

The very first time I ever read about penis-enlargement surgery was in July 1991, when the UK's newspaper the *Sun* published an article with the eye-catching headline of 'Hello, Bigger Boy!' My previous book fills in all the details.

Here I will give a layman's opinion and general details about the quite-varied ways a man's penis can be enlarged surgically.

The first surgeon I will mention, therefore, is Dr Harold Reed, who is the doctor mentioned in the *Sun's* article I discuss above. For my research in writing this book, I contacted Dr Reed by e-mail. He informed me that he has been performing penile enlargement operations since 1986, and he has completed 'well over three thousand' phalloplasty (penoplasty) procedures.

The photographic gallery on his website shows some of the penises he has operated on, and it's a real eye-opener. There's the guy I called 'Big Wood' for obvious reasons. I've often imagined what it would be like to have a penis as big as that just for one day. The trouble is, I wouldn't want to give it back to the owner! I've also noticed a man in his gallery who has undergone girth enhancement, and the photo shows his penis fully erect—his hand can only get about halfway around his manhood.

Reading Dr Reed's website, it's interesting to see that he prefers to perform the lengthening and thickening operations as two completely different procedures. Apparently he feels that he achieves better results by doing separate operations. Most other surgeons around the world seem to perform the procedures on the same day.

On his website he explains that penis-lengthening techniques (or phalloplasty) have been described in urological literature for at least forty years. The procedure involves, as needed, release of the suspensory ligament, pubic liposuction or dissection and taking down the 'turkey neck' (peno-scrotal web).

Dr Reed says that well-motivated patients who follow his postoperative instructions have achieved length gains of up to two inches. Furthermore he explains that his postoperative regimen centres on the use of The Grip system for penile traction.

As for penile girth, Dr Reed states this can be performed by one of three techniques:

a) Placement of dermal-fat grafts which are harvested from the lower abdomen or buttocks area,

b) Insertion of Alloderm strips, or

c) Insertion of liposuctioned fat

For more detailed information you can visit his website or his blog which lists *all* the procedures he performs as well as the costs of each operation.

I obviously cannot personally vouch for his skills as a surgeon because I haven't 'gone under the knife' with Dr Reed. That said, considering he's been performing penile enlargement since 1986, I would find it hard to believe there are many surgeons around with more experience in this field than Dr Reed. I have to say his before-and-after gallery of enhanced penises is impressive, to put it mildly.

Regarding penis enlargement surgery in Britain and Europe, I think for expertise we do not have to look any further than Dr Roberto Viel at the London Centre for Aesthetic Surgery. He is based in the United Kingdom, along with his twin, Maurizio, at 15 Harley Street, London, London, W1G 9QQ; the telephone number is +44(0)207636 4272. The Centre's website is www.lcas.com, and the e-mail address is info@lcas.com. They have been performing penile enlargement procedures since 1991.

On the introduction to the clinic's website, they state the following: 'Penile size can be significantly enhanced in both length and width without affecting sexual performance or sensitivity by the well-established surgical techniques called penoplasty'.

They go on to say that penoplasty is justified when the psychological benefits outweigh the risk and cost of the procedure.

The detailed recommendations listed on the site under 'Before Your Penile Enlargement Surgery' are as follows: 'In the week before (the operation) you should not take any medications containing aspirin (acetyl salicylic acid), since these products affect the blood clotting mechanism and therefore may lead to excessive bleeding during and after surgery, hence resulting in increased bruising. Taking high doses of vitamin E preparations, eating large amounts of garlic and consuming alcohol can also produce the same result and should be avoided. If pain medication is necessary, we recommend you take ibuprofen/paracetamol'.

One absolute must is to quit smoking at least two weeks before and up to two weeks after surgery. It is well known that smoking causes a narrowing of the blood vessels, which leads to decreased blood supply to the skin, thus slowing and interfering with the healing process. I'm a good boy, as I haven't smoked for at least twenty-five years or more. The cigarettes I did smoke, I deeply regret. Dr Horn explained that one of the reasons I didn't have any bruising to speak of is that I don't smoke. Let that be a warning to *all* you smokers out there.

The above information is then followed by 'The Penoplasty Procedure at LCAS London'. 'To increase the length, an incision will be made above the base of the penis. Through this, we can release the penile suspensory ligament, thus allowing the penis to be brought forward, thereby lengthening it externally by typically one to two inches. Men with prominent pubic fat pads will gain more length; if, for example, they have a two-inch fat pad, and one and a half inches is removed, the additional one-and-a-half-inch gain will be supplemental to the extension gained by releasing the suspensory ligament.

'The increase in girth involves a small amount of liposuction of the stomach or thigh areas to collect fat, followed by reintroduction of the fat by injection along the shaft of the penis. The usual increase in girth is between one to two inches. The fat-injection procedure avoids incision scars and because it is a simpler technique, the recovery time is shorter.'

Then we are told the following details: 'Penoplasty is a day-case procedure, and will be performed at our Harley Street clinic under local anaesthetic with IV sedation (this is not a general anaesthetic). You will be completely pain free and will not remember anything about the procedure.' I find this part *very* interesting.

We then reach the section 'After the Procedure': 'In the case of lengthening, you will have deep-dissolving sutures in the underlying muscle and tissue and some skin sutures as well as staples to the pubis. With the enlargement, you will have only one small suture to the abdomen (where we collected the fat) and one further suture to the base of the penis (where the fat was injected), as well as some strapping across the abdomen for one week. You will remain at the clinic for about two hours, to allow us to monitor your recovery from the sedation.'

Patients of Dr Viel are informed that, after two or three days following the surgery, they may experience a slight amount of discomfort, but this is normally controlled with oral pain relief. Patients are also warned that they may experience a small amount of bruising and some surgical swelling, which will subside after approximately two weeks. Massaging of the penis using Vaseline is recommended each day to resolve the asymmetry of the penis and to prevent lumps from occurring.

A week after the operation, patients will return to the clinic to have bandages and sutures removed. Further visits to the clinic will be required to ensure that the healing process is proceeding satisfactory. Sexual activity can normally be resumed after one month, however it can take three to six months to achieve the maximum length gained from elongation.

A warning is given to prospective patients: 'Like all operations, penoplasty is not without complications. They are rare but can occur. These include infection, bleeding, and blood under the skin, known as haematoma or blood clot; however this occurs in less than 1 percent of patients and drains and heals spontaneously.'

From Harley Street in London I will now go back to the United States, specifically to California and New York. The surgeon in question is Dr Gary J. Alter, MD, who specialises in penis and scrotal surgery.

Within his expertise is performing operations on men who suffer from hidden or buried penis. His website explains as follows:

A hidden penis is frequently referred to as a buried or concealed penis. There are multiple causes of buried penis including obesity, aging with an overlying fold of abdominal fat and skin, and a shortage of penile skin from chronic inflammation or an overly aggressive circumcision.

Some men are born with a congenital fat pad that tends to make the penis inconspicuous. The skin of the lower abdomen and pubis descends or sags with age, causing the penis of some men to hide under the excess skin and fat. Obesity makes the concealment of the penis worse. Various procedures are available to make the penis more visible if the penile shaft is buried below the surface of the skin from obesity or aging, an overly aggressive circumcision, congenital fat deposits, or a small phallus.

If excess skin and fat are present on the lower abdomen and pubis, the skin and fat are excised, elevating the pubic region and giving a more youthful appearance to the penis and genitalia. If fat only is present, liposuction or open surgical removal of the fat is performed. The skin of the pubis is sutured down to the underlying abdominal tissue, which prevents the penis from hiding in the pubic area. The skin at the base of the penis and scrotum is sutured to the erectile bodies, preventing the penis from retracting into fat or into the scrotum.

The extent of the operation depends on the severity of the deformity. Surgery is usually done as an outpatient. The improvement in penile and pubic appearance can be dramatic.

Men suffering from a hidden or buried penis who have any questions are invited to contact Board Certified Plastic Surgeon, Board Certified Urologist Dr Gary Alter at his Manhattan, New York or Beverly Hills, California office.

I would definitely recommend you visit Dr Alter's website, where you can see his excellent work he's performed on men who have a hidden or buried penis. Excellent work indeed. I defy *any* agony aunt, therapist, doctor, psychiatrist, or psychotherapist to say that penis size doesn't matter. The men shown on the website cannot urinate properly, never mind normal have sexual intercourse. If you don't believe me, please look at the website—it may not be something you would show your favourite Aunt but at least you may understand the trauma that these men go through.

If you are American, British, or any other nationality and you are unfortunate enough to suffer from this terrible affliction, please get in touch with Dr Alter at altermd@altermd.com if you want help. I know it will cost money, but many good things aren't free. The website says,

'Prices for different cosmetic procedures are determined by the operation necessary.' Not every man will have the money, but at least it's worth saving up for.

Dr Alter's addresses are as follows: 416 North Bedford Drive, Suite 400, Beverly Hills, CA 90210, phone: (310) 275-5566; and 461 Park Avenue South, Seventh Floor, New York, NY 10016, phone: (310) 275-5566.

American surgeons perform more penoplasty procedures and, of course, there are practitioners in the United States. I will try to inform you of the most-experienced ones.

One such surgeon is Dr E. Douglas Whitehead, MD, FACS who is based at 24 East 12th Street, Suite 2-1, New York, NY 10003, Tel: 1-800-575-1112 (International: +212-620 5308), e-mail: info@drwhitehead.com. When I last saw his website, there were many before-and-after photos for you to look at. As always, if you want to ask him questions, then go ahead and ask him. If you want to speak to one or more of his patients that have undergone penoplasty don't be shy to ask him or his staff. You owe it to yourself.

There is also Dr Mark P. Solomon MD, FACS, who has two locations. One is based at 30 Central Park South, Tenth Floor, New York, NY 10019 (Phone: 347-922-8882), and the other at his Philadelphia Office, 191 Presidential Boulevard Suite, LN 24 Bala Cynwyd, PA 19004 (Phone: 610-667-7070).

He has been performing surgery for twenty-six years and has rejected 30 percent of prospective patients due to their 'unrealistic expectations'. I applaud that attitude because the last thing a reputable surgeon wants is a disappointed patient who thinks the surgeon can perform miracles. No such surgeon exists.

Another very experienced surgeon, Dr R. S. Barron, runs the Barron Centers at 465 N. Roxbury Drive # 1012, Beverly Hills, CA 90210, Phone: 1-800-372-6990 and e-mail: info@thebarroncenters.com. Dr Barron was certified by the American Board of Urology in 1985, the same year he established his practice in Beverly Hills. Due to the increasing number of men Dr Barron saw in his practice in the late 1980s requesting penile enlargement, he began his efforts to develop penile enlargement procedures. He has continued to develop and refine the procedures and receives requests from physicians from all parts of the world who want to learn his techniques.

I will now relate something to you all about a Canadian surgeon, Dr Robert H. Stubbs, who has performed over one thousand penoplasty procedures. His interest in this operation began when he read about Dr Long, Professor of Plastic Surgery, in Wuhan, China. In 1984, a young man who had his penis bitten off by a dog during infancy asked Dr Long if he could lengthen his penis so that he could marry. A reconstructive procedure using plastic surgical techniques was performed successfully. Dr Long was then able to offer his knowledge and skill to cosmetic patients who, although 'normal', were unhappy with their size. Dr Stubbs visited Dr Long in 1993. After returning to Canada, he modified and improved the technique for the more 'demanding' North American male.

There are a great number of surgeons and clinics in Europe—both eastern and western—who perform penile enlargement surgery. Really all you would have to do is type into your computer 'penis enlargement surgery Italy/Germany/France/Romania/Poland' or any other European country that interests you and the details will become available. If you're without a computer you could always contact me via Create Space, and I could give you the details you require.

What really interested me was looking at penis-enlargement surgery in India, which has a vast male population. On one Indian website there's understandably the following headline—'Penis Enlargement'. The introduction continues, 'There has always been a great demand for penile enlargement and dissatisfaction about the length and the girth of the penis in each individual. Many men desire greater length and the thickness of the penis. It is important for any individual to understand the procedure for the penile enlargement before submitting themselves for these procedures with great expectations. It is for these men to understand that though procedures are available and successful but they are meant for the "Needy but not for the Greedy"'. This clinic sounds good to me because they stress any prospective patients should have realistic expectations. Consider the clinic's message—'Needy but not for the Greedy'.

Now let's turn to the other Asian country with a huge male population, namely China. One website that caught my eye was 'China Cosmetic Surgery, Shenyang, China'. Concerning penis enlargement surgery, it was written there, 'Approximately one-third to one-half of the penis is inside the body, it is attached to the under surface of the pubic bone by suspension ligaments. The result of surgically releasing these ligaments brings more of the penis outside the body providing more functional length.'

According to the figures quoted, in 2014 the cost of the combined procedures—lengthening and thickening—amounts to $1,875. The address for the clinic is: China Cosmetic Surgery, 28 Renao Road, Shenyang City, Liaoning Province China 110014. The e-mail address is: info@china–cosmetic-surgery.com.

For my last surgeon in this particular chapter, I'm going to return to the United Kingdom. It may be no surprise that I'm going to mention, and recommend, Dr Gary Horn. He has performed my last two penoplasty operations, which entailed harvesting fat from my buttocks to enhance my girth. I swear on my daughter's life that I was very happy with the results. I didn't expect the world, but I would say that's good enough for me.

You will see from reading the Mayfair Clinic's website how the procedure is undertaken. The increase in girth is achieved by harvesting fat from the patient's abdomen or buttocks. This procedure can increase the girth by one to three inches. My own opinion is that it helps if the patient has some surplus fat which can produce sufficiently good reserves to top-up further girth enhancement.

There is, however, a variant of the fat-transfer method called 'dermal transfer'. Dermal transfer uses strips of skin and fat together. The skin stops the fat from being reabsorbed into the body.

The lengthening procedure is explained as follows, 'The tissue in the penis that fills with blood is called the *corpora cavernosa*. This spongy tissue normally extends from the penis back into the body. Half of the *corpora cavernosa* may be "concealed" inside the body. Penis lengthening relies on releasing this concealed tissue, which has the effect of increasing the visible length of the penis. Releasing the concealed part of the penis is done by cutting the suspensory ligaments that keep the *corpora cavernosa* anchored within the body. This moves the concealed part of the penis forward achieving additional penis length outside the body.'

The details continue on the Mayfair Clinic's website as follows:

Aim

The aim of the operation is to permanently lengthen the penis by three centimetres (one and a half inches).

Swelling

This varies, but yes, following your operation you will have some swelling but usually this subsides after about one week.

Bruising

Yes, this varies from one person to another.

Recovery

The decision about when to return to work and resume normal activities depends on how fast you heal and how well you feel. As a general guide it is usual for clients to return to work after about ten to fourteen days.

Final Result Visible

Although an improvement may be seen almost immediately it may take up to three months to see the final result.

Can the Penis Girth Be Enlarged at the Same Time?

Most clients do opt for the thickness procedure to be performed at the same time as the lengthening operation.

We greatly value our customers and believe in offering informed, educated personal guidance every step of the way. Before you make the choice to undergo any treatment or solution, we invite you for an initial complimentary consultation in the luxurious privacy of the Mayfair Clinic.

Reading this, it does make one wonder how the man, mentioned in chapter one, who underwent the penoplasty procedure at the Mayfair Clinic, should be so naive and totally lacking in understanding of the advice and aftercare he was given.

From my personal experience of Dr Horn's surgical skills and Anna Camilleri's ability as a cosmetic consultant, I certainly have no hesitation in recommending them should you wish to undergo penoplasty at the Mayfair Clinic.

I would just add that any man going to the clinic for this operation should heed the advice and be realistic regarding the initial results from their first operation.

CHAPTER FOUR

New Techniques for Penoplasty

Since I had my first and most major penoplasty in August 1996, many new surgical and nonsurgical techniques have evolved to both lengthen and thicken a man's penis.

I discovered a description of a new method of penile enlargement. The heading was 'Penis enlargement: ventral and dorsal combined technique.' Looking at my dictionary this quite simply means front (ventral) and back (dorsal) of the penis.

At the second Ibero-American Conference of Andrology in December 2003, the following aspects of penis enlargement were discussed:

The Koro Syndrome:

'Small penis syndrome, which provokes psychological disorders affecting one's personality and social behaviour, although it is not to be considered a psychiatric disease.'

The Changing Room Syndrome:

The problem arises because of the look of one's own penis in the state of flaccidity. Two-thirds of men accept the way their penis looks. The rest prefer hiding it, although they report no problem in having sexual intercourse.

Such set of syndromes is worsened by the following factors: the way or angle one looks at one's penis, malicious remarks or jokes from one's friends or partner, and the spread of pornography.

Penis Enlargement, the Combined Technique:

Average penis size, taken from the pubis to the glans in the state of flaccidity and under traction, varies between ten and fourteen centimetres. The size of the majority of people is normal, and so is their erectile function.

It should be noted this is *not* just another plastic surgery technique. We are called upon to ask ourselves whether the results can be positive, what are the best techniques, whether the quality of sexual intercourse is satisfactory, and what the side effects can be.

Ethics of results: completely satisfactory results cannot be reached, and the patient cannot have all his expectations fulfilled.

Noninvasive Procedures:

Vacuum pumps (totally ineffective)

Andropenis: mechanism of continuous traction that gives real enlargement.

Surgical Procedures:

First surgery: Dr Long 1984

Various techniques exist, though they all include the following:

Snipping of the suspensory ligament,

Separation of the fundiform ligaments, and

Suprapubic liposuction (in some cases).

Surgical Techniques:

Balanopreputial incision,

Penis denudation to the base of the shaft,

Snipping and ligation of the superficial dorsal vein,
Snipping of the suspensory ligament, and
Snipping of the fundiform ligaments.

A constant traction of the penis shaft during surgery is advisable to ease the ligament snipping, establish the actual elongation, and precisely carry out the lateral ligation of the *albuginea* to the straight abdominal terminal membrane, thus impeding penile retraction.

A rigorous *hemostasis* is necessary. Total bandaging for the first ten days is advisable. The Andropenis is to be worn three to four weeks after surgery for no less than two months.

Postsurgical Recovery:

Anti-inflammatory drugs for ten days. Varbiotic every eight hours for five days. Keep bandaging on for ten days. Local cold applications in the first hours after surgery.

Main Complications:

Bruising, penile retraction, oedema, loss of sensitivity, and psychogenic erectile functions.

Our Experience:

Twenty-five patients who had unique combined techniques experienced an average gain in length of five centimetres. No complications. High degree of satisfaction for most patients.

Another new technique I discovered when researching this book was under the heading: 'Length-boosting surgery for "micropenises"'.

The details were explained as follows:
A new surgical procedure has allowed men with abnormally short penises to enjoy a full sex life and urinate standing up, some for the first time. Tiny 'micropenises' have been enlarged

to normal size without losing any erogenous sensation, say UK doctors.

'Micropenis' refers to any penis shorter than seven centimetres when fully erect—approximately half of the average length (twelve and a half centimetres).

Approximately one in every two hundred men have a micro-penis, either because of a birth defect or because they have undergone cancer treatments.

'It's not so much penile enlargement as penile construction', says David Ralph at the University College of London, United Kingdom, who will describe the technique on Wednesday at a sexual medicine conference in London. Until now, these men have not been able to have sex or urinate because their penis was too short.

In the past, flaps of skin from the forearm had been used to reconstruct a penis from scratch, either to physically transform women into men or to replace an amputated penis. But this technique actually fuses the new penis with the existing one so, besides the adding of sheer bulk, erogenous sensation can be preserved.

Cylindrical flap

Ralph operated on nine men aged between nineteen and forty-three with a range of medical histories, including three hermaphrodites, two with other birth defects and two whose penises did not develop properly after undergoing chemotherapy as infants.

He made three twelve-and-a-half-centimetre incisions in the arms of these patients, harvesting a square flap of skin. While it was still attached to the arm he rolled it up like 'a Swiss roll' with a tube running down the centre. Ralph then cut off the cylindrical flap and sewed it at one end to the base of the micropenis—so that the original penis ran along the inside of the cylinder.

New Techniques for Penoplasty

To preserve erogenous sensation, he also cut the tip of the penis—called the glans—away from the main shaft, while leaving the blood vessels and nerves intact. While still being connected to the blood vessels and nerves of the micropenis, the glans was sewn back to the outside end of the new penis. Arteries, veins and nerves from the pelvis were also joined to supply the new penis.

Full sexual function

The skin on the arm is perfect, says Ralph, because the blood vessels are about the same size as those in the pelvis and are positioned so that the two can easily be joined together. The arm is restored with a skin graft from the buttocks.

But for full sexual function, a penile prosthesis—used frequently by men who have problems achieving an erection—must also be implanted. It consists of a silicone cylinder that lines the penis shaft and is attached via a pump to a silicone reservoir in the abdomen. Pushing a button under the scrotum causes fluid to pass from the reservoir into the shaft, stiffening the penis.

'It's certainly a nice gain for the field', says Anthony Atala, a urologist at Wake Forest School of Urology in Winston-Salam, North Carolina, United States of America. 'No one had ever combined the disconnection of the glans with a skin graft', he says.

Another absolutely sensational story regarding penile enlargement/ penile reconstruction was reported in the *Sun* on February 27 and 28, 2013. The report on February 27 caught my attention with the headline 'Docs to rebuild hubby's lost willy'. Mohammed Abad was interviewed on ITV1'S *This Morning* when he informed Philip Schofield and Holly Willoughby about an accident when he was six. He fell under a car and was dragged six hundred feet, losing his penis and a testicle.

Mohammed told his incredible story to the watching public how he was given just twelve hours to live but doctors saved him and created a penis so he could go to the toilet. However, it had no sexual function later in life. Sadly his parents never explained he would not have any children and how severe his problem would be.

The story continued in the *Sun* the next day with the extremely eye-catching headline, 'My Willy Is Made out of My Arm'. He had appeared on channel four's medical show *Embarrassing Bodies,* where consultant uroandrolgists Mr Nim Christopher and Mr David Ralph performed an incredible operation on his genitals.

The consultants rebuilt his manhood with fat taken from his arm. More accurately the consultants cut two six-inch grafts from his left arm, which affectively gave him a six-inch appendage! The operation was shown not only on *Embarrassing Bodies* but also on *This Morning.*

Viewers on *This Morning* were warned about the film, which would show parts of the operation along with Mohammed's newly rebuilt penis. Along with Philip, Holly, and Mohammed was Dr Chris Steele who explained certain technical and surgical aspects of the procedure.

Dr Steele noted how large Mohammed's penis is—being six inches when only soft. It was also acknowledged how very thick his penis was. The pioneering surgery, which involved a twelve-hour operation, was performed at the University College London in late 2012 when his new penis was formed, 'like a Swiss roll'.

Mohammed had an arranged marriage a couple of years ago, but his new wife had been unaware of his accident and that he had no real penis to speak of. Although she refused to be named she was 100 percent in favour of the operation.

Both TV programmes showed his initial consultation with Mr Christopher, when it was explained that skin grafts would be taken from his arm to reconstruct his penis. Mr Christopher explained that Mohammed had large arms and that this would mean his penis could be made to be about six inches in length as well as being thick. Needless to say, Mohammed was delighted to hear this.

CHAPTER FIVE

Botched Penoplasty Jobs

Unfortunately, particularly in the early days of penis enlargement surgery, there were some really awful operations that went horrifically wrong.

The television documentary that I appeared on in 2004 showed horrific photographs of penile enlargement operations that went horribly wrong. I don't know where the producer obtained the photographs, but they were definitely rated X. Even adults would feel queasy after looking at such botched operations.

I know when I wrote my first book that I had to mention a certain American surgeon by the name of Dr Melvyn Rosenstein, otherwise known as Dr Dick, who boasted he had performed between five thousand to seven thousand penoplasty (phalloplasty) procedures. He was, according to his office, performing the procedure on between five to ten men a day. That's an awful lot of surgery, and perhaps the more surgeries he performed, the higher the chances that he got things horribly wrong. This is not good news for the poor guys that end up with misshapen and infected penises.

A number of patients ended up with infected, deformed, or just plain badly swollen penises. Some men, it was alleged, ended up with impotence. I simply don't know what the true numbers are. There may have been dozens or hundreds of men unable to function sexually after

MICROPENIS: The Long and Short of It

Dr Rosenstein had finished off his handiwork. The problem is that there may have been some men jumping on the bandwagon in an effort to prosecute the surgeon for millions of dollars. Or maybe not, perhaps only the men involved know the true scale of their problems.

Don't get me wrong. If a man has been left with impotence or with a badly infected penis, he deserves to get every penny he can get his hands on. Hopefully, he could then get the mess cleared up by a far better and more-honest surgeon and clinic.

There's no doubt that any negligent and greedy surgeon should have his licence revoked and be made to pay any compensation to the poor men he so badly operated on.

The only thing I would say is that occasionally there are people who seek compensation when none should be forthcoming. Some people act innocent when there's chance of a fast buck. As mentioned earlier in chapter one, some men have totally unrealistic expectations regarding the first operation. They may want to ignore some of the sensible advice the surgeon, clinic or nursing staff have given them.

If the surgeon is totally at fault, then let's throw the book at him (or her). Hopefully you, the reader, agree with me on that point. They should be held to account for any of their wrongdoings.

When I wrote my first book, the female producer of *Drastic Plastic* suggested I should write a piece warning men about the possible pit-falls of unscrupulous surgeons and/or clinics. Some clinics, even to-day, will try to offer you the earth and yet provide you with as little aftercare as possible. This should be a no-no for patients who have invested a lot of time, energy, hope, and money in having an operation they have probably longed for over many years. To be let down so badly after waiting such a long time to have the operation must be really heart-breaking.

If you saw *Drastic Plastic* on channel five, you would know that some men's penises ended up being horribly infected and misshapen after surgery. We are not talking about minor problems; we are now talking about problems on a major scale. Any man unfortunate enough to receive this abysmal treatment does deserve to receive financial compensation. This, of course, does not give them back a healthy penis (whether it's big, small, or tiny), but at least such men will get their money back and then some. Further surgery to make good the mistakes will hopefully be undertaken by a skilled surgeon.

I know for certain there has been a penoplasty operation that ended in a fatality. The cosmetic surgeon was Dr Ricardo Samitier, who was convicted of manslaughter after a man he operated on bled to death in May 1992. The patient concerned was Claudio Martell, who went to Dr Samitier to reduce his double chin, chubby cheeks, and tighten his pot belly, as well as have his penis enlarged.

Tragically, Mr Martell had an enlarged heart and a pacemaker, and he took blood-thinning medication. During the operation Dr Samitier could not stop the patient's bleeding and was not equipped to treat Mr Martell's heart when it stopped beating.

Dr Samitier received a five-year prison sentence. He had already lost his medical licence in January 1992. The patient tragically lost his life.

I know this is an extreme example, but any person considering cosmetic surgery must be aware of all the risks. I think some surgeons who perform penile enlargement operations are not trained sufficiently to perform some of these procedures.

A story that caught my eye for all the wrong reasons was a report in the *Guardian* on July 12, 2011, entitled 'Backstreet Botch-Up'. The article explained that in 2009, one million, one hundred thousand nonsurgical procedures were performed and that in March 2011 Superdrug became the first high-street retailer to offer budget antiwrinkle injections, derma-fillers, and other treatments that are usually the preserve of private clinics.

According to Fazel Fatah, consultant plastic surgeon and president of the British Association of Aesthetic Plastic Surgeons, 'The notion that people call "aesthetic treatments" has been developed around various injectables and noninvasive procedures. This has allowed people with no medical training to establish a practice and make easy money with little, if any, thought as to the patients' wellbeing.'

The article went on to explain that the organisation is particularly worried about backstreet procedures for men seeking genital enhancements. It said that there is evidence of a number of websites promoting the use of silicone injections in scrotums and penises—unlicensed treatments performed by medically unqualified practitioners that can result in serious medical problems.

A fifty-year-old aircraft engineer, Jim Horton, underwent one such procedure in 2007. He had always wanted a bigger scrotum, and when he started scanning various online chat sites, he realised he could get it done rather cheaply. Jim e-mailed a guy who seemed very professional and above-board.

It was only when he arrived for his appointment that Jim began to worry. 'I thought there'd be some kind of surgery inside—but it was nothing more than a normal house.' It became apparent that the 'surgeon', or whatever he called himself, actually claimed to work on some North Sea oil rigs. The man claimed to have done this procedure on more than ninety men as well as having had silicone injected into his own penis and scrotum. Jim trusted him and they went upstairs.

But after Jim had showered and was lying on the bed, waiting to be injected, things started to go wrong. 'I noticed the silicone was kept in an open milk bottle on the side—and this guy put the syringe full of the silicone into a regular sealant gun you'd buy from a DIY store. He said he needed to apply extra pressure as the fluid was so thick, but by now I was in his hands and went along with it.'

Over the next thirty minutes, Jim had sixty millilitres of silicone injected into each side of his scrotum. Afterwards, he got dressed and handed over £120. 'I felt fine, and my scrotum looked and felt better. I was happy with what I'd paid for', Jim reported to the *Guardian*.

Botched Penoplasty Jobs

However, by Christmas, he noticed that the injected areas had started to harden and become misshapen. Jim phoned the guy, asking if this was normal, and he just said, 'Bad luck', and then he hung up. Jim felt very stupid and angry for having put himself in such a position.

Over the next eighteen months, Jim's problems got worse as the silicone hardened around his testicles—it felt like they had been burdened with a weight. Jim couldn't sleep and couldn't work, and he felt like a freak. Finally, in February 2010, he met a consultant urologist in Bristol, who tried to remove the silicone in an operation.

Unfortunately, the operation had to be stopped when the flesh on his scrotum lost its blood supply. Jim spent the next three weeks at home with a district nurse coming round every day to dress the wound and to keep it clean. Jim remarked rather angrily that the 'smell of rotting flesh was absolutely horrendous.'

Next, the consultant urologist and a cosmetic surgeon took a skin graft from his leg to replace the skin on his scrotum. It was explained to Jim that they couldn't get the silicone out without risking cutting off vital blood supplies, but they could sort out his scrotum.

Regrettably, after the operation, the skin tightened, leaving Jim in agony. He was admitted as an emergency case in April 2012 when the urologist and cosmetic surgeon removed 80 percent of the silicone. Within a week, Jim was readmitted to hospital with an infection and was then on a drip for four days.

Happily, Jim's wounds have now healed, and he feels almost human for the first time in five years. He said he was relieved to be able to walk and function again, and he expressed his thanks to the surgeons and the NHS who had helped him get over the stupid mess he had created for himself.

Jim's final words were, 'I just want to expose this backstreet industry and stop other men going down the same route I did.'

That is a pretty gruesome story and one which should be told to any man considering this 'backstreet' enhancement procedure. No man could have been more desperate than me, having a micropenis, but even

MICROPENIS: The Long and Short of It

I would have not resorted to having silicone injected into my penis with a sealant gun.

Another appalling story appeared on the Internet, concerning a twenty-two-year-old man who had died after having a so-called penis-enlargement procedure. Police in New Jersey, America, arrested a woman on charges of homicide after she allegedly used silicone injections to increase the size of Justin Street's penis. The thirty-four-year-old woman, Ms Kasia Rivera, was also charged with the illegal practice of medicine, which resulted in a blood clot that killed the patient. The surgical injections were said to have been carried out in the home of Ms Rivera.

A story is currently on the Internet (as of 2014) that again stretches the imagination, to put it mildly. Under the heading, 'Trying Desperately to Measure Up', a story is told that doctors in Asia are treating an increasing number of men with severe injuries who have tried to increase the size of their penises by injecting themselves with Vaseline and other oils. Now doctors in the West say the trend for self-injection is catching on in the United Kingdom and in the United States.

Injuries consist of severe deformations caused by tissue damage and erectile dysfunction. Gangrene can also develop if the injection causes an infection. According to Mr Manit Arya, a urologist at the Institute of Urology and Nephrology (IUN) in London, 'Increasing the size of the girth of the penis is common in Southeast Asia as well as in Japan.'

So for men who want to increase their sizes, particularly their girth, please do not start injecting your penis with Vaseline or any other oil-based material. In fact, don't inject your penis with any substance—go to an experienced surgeon qualified to perform penile enlargement.

To those other men it must be said: Never consider a backstreet shyster, because that's why he or she 'performs' these awful procedures in a dark and dingy back room. Don't ever forget these people are potentially 'performing' lethal procedures.

I know I'm repeating myself *ad nauseam*, but if you want penis enlargement, please go to a reputable surgeon. You know it makes sense.

CHAPTER SIX

Size Queens

Well, there's no beating about the bush: many women do prefer well-endowed men, and that's a fact. My supposition is that most men know it—and certainly the majority of women know it, even if some women tread carefully, saying that a woman loves the man, not the penis. There is a limit to this particular cliché, and to be honest, I find it condescending in the extreme. Fancy a woman saying to a man, 'Don't worry, darling, I love your personality, your caring, compassionate ways, and your generosity, but I don't really care about your penis.' Talk about a backhanded compliment!

You will find dozens of examples in my first book where women admit publicly that they prefer larger men—they are not shallow; they are just being honest. Does it make them better women if they trot out the same old phrases as, 'It's not the size, it's what you do with it'? As a man who suffered from micropenis, I just want to scream, 'Give me a break, please!'

What did Robert Plant mean when he was singing (shouting?) on the song 'Whole Lotta Love', 'I wanna give you every inch of my love'? For goodness' sake, we know he was not talking about his shirt collar size.

MICROPENIS: The Long and Short of It

The following examples regarding size queens have found their way onto the Internet:

1. Mamie Van Doren: 'In my autobiography, *Playing the Field*, I was one of the first celebrities to openly discuss the penis sizes of the men I knew. Because of that, the book caused quite a stir in its day. Talk show hosts, especially men, were very intimidated by a woman who frankly evaluated men the way men had evaluated women over the years—by inches. I once said that seven and a half inches was the ideal penis size for me. What, you may ask, is the basis for such a specific measurement? It is a complicated equation, to be sure—part astrology, part East Indian Karma Sutra, and part old-fashioned carpenter's tape measure. And experience. It's the scientific method: experimentation. Go figure. It's the right size.'

2. Sarah Silverman: 'Does size matter? Yes. My rabbi sister is going to kill me about this, but even she said that if her husband didn't have a big dick they would just be friends. Next question.'

3. Janice Dickinson had this to say about Mick Jagger, with whom she had a relationship in the 1980s: 'He has the smallest penis alive. He's nasty little Sir Mick with a little dick. It was very little.' This isn't the first time she has disparaged the size of Mick's member. A couple of years ago, I think, she was on Jonathon Ross in the United Kingdom and held up her pinky. She said at the time that her pinky would have been an improvement. As for a celebrity who is well endowed, she chose Liam Neeson. 'He took his pants off, and an Evian bottle fell out. It was huge.'

4. Fergie: 'I think women are beautiful. I've had a lot of fun with women, and I'm not ashamed of it. The problem is that I also love well-endowed men.'

5. Sarah Brightman was asked on a UK talk show by Graham Norton about why she went out with Andrew Lloyd Webber. 'Because he simply has the *biggest* penis', she replied.

6. Janet Jackson: 'I'm a size queen. Honestly, if I'm on a date and I see the guy is not packing, that's when I fake a backache. Suddenly, your back goes out. I learned that from my friends. Hmmm... what constitutes a nice package in my opinion? A pretty good size. I've been called a size queen before. My friends tease me about it. I just like nice packages. A god-size package.' What does that mean? 'Honestly he's gotta be hangin'.' When the writer says he thought the song's term refers to other qualities about a guy, she corrects him. 'No. No, It's just about one thing. It's about the kickstand, that's all...It's a girly thing. When girlfriends get together, they talk about guys just the way guys get together and talk about girls.' When the writer asked, 'You talk about size?' Ms Jackson replied, 'Well, you know? We talk about you guys. Who's big, who's not. We talk about a lot of things. Sorry.'

7. Linda Fiorentino: When asked what she looks for in the men she's attracted to, she said, 'Intelligence. Sense of humour. And a big cock. That's it. In that order. A nerd with a big penis. Ideal. A genius with a penis. Isn't that we all want? I go to bed with men, not boys.' When asked what women want these days, she said, 'Sometimes all we need is a big dick and no arguments. What could make us happier?' Her interviewer asked, 'Isn't that a bit simplistic?' She replied, 'Maybe, but I've learned not to expect that much in relationships. So being well hung is at least compensation for a general lack of sensitivity in the emotional area.'

8. Heidi Klum informed Oprah Winfrey on a show yet to air that it wasn't Seal's music that caused her to fall for him. The sight of him in spandex shorts sealed the deal. 'When I saw him, I was like, wow! He is different and so tall and dark and just handsome. I saw the package—and I mean the whole package, literally. I was like, "That is a man."'

9. Keeley Hazell, when she was asked, 'What's the very first thing you notice on a guy when it's just lust at first sight? Be honest!'

answered, 'His trouser bulge! Hey, you told me to be honest. It's no good getting close to a guy and then finding out he can't deliver the goods. Size *does* matter. Although you know that, don't you!'

10. Pamela Anderson: 'I'm not going to pretend it doesn't make a difference. I know some women say that size doesn't matter. But it does, at least for me. Put it this way, I can't see any down side to a man being well hung. So many women fight over how big their diamonds are, but the size of the stone is really about their man's ego over his little thing. I think diamonds have a direct relationship to your man's penis size. Does size count? Unfortunately, yes. Size definitely matters. Whoever says size doesn't matter is a liar with a small dick. But I'm lucky I never met any of those.'

11. Michelle Branch, when interviewed in the January issue of *Maxim* magazine, recalled that when she met a giant NFL player with 'huge, beautiful hands', she desperately wanted 'to see what's in his pants! Can you imagine what it must be like?'

12. Courtney Cox said on Howard Stern's radio show that penis size was important to her.

13. Molly Culver, when on the *Howard Stern Show*, agreed with Pamela Anderson that penis size is very important. She claimed to be able to pick out a well-endowed man from a crowd. Stern had the guys in the studio line up, and she correctly picked out the one with the biggest penis.

14. Kimberly 'Lil' Kim' Jones, in her song 'How Many Licks', talked about one of her favourite lovers. 'And this black dude I called King Kong/He had a big-ass dick and a hurricane tongue.' In her collaboration with the notorious Tommy Lee, 'Methods of Mayhem', she rapped 'Under seven inches? Eh, sorry, minimen. I can't fuck with them.'

15. Rihanna, when asked by German magazine *Bravo* what a guy needed to impress her, she replied, 'He has to be good in bed, and the size matters. You know what I mean?'

16. Josie Maran said, 'I'm really shallow when I come to guys. I only date really good-looking, well-endowed guys with great bodies. My friends are always going on at me. I'm like, "I can't help it! I'm just a woman with high standards!"'

Last, but certainly not least, when Lady Gaga was asked what men she preferred, she answered without hesitation, 'It ranges from a really big dick to a degree at Harvard.'

I did overhear a young, attractive woman discuss penis size with other women. She explained that if she had a choice between two men who were very attractive and who both had wonderful personalities, she would find it very difficult to make a choice on which one she would like to have as her boyfriend. However, if she discovered one had a micropenis (three inches or less and very thin in girth), and the other guy was well hung (seven or eight inches and thick in girth), she would undoubtedly choose the well-hung guy.

In the issue of the *Sun* dated April 9, 2013, an article entitled 'Girls Size Up Guys' reported that 'Size really does matter when attracting a woman.' A study undertaken by biologist Dr Brian Mautz reported that more than one hundred women were shown computer-generated images of naked men—and preferred those with a bigger willy.

Dr Mautz, who did this research in Canberra, Australia, suggested that penis size is as important to a man's attractiveness as his stature. The report also discovered that having greater shoulder-to-hip ratio also influenced desirability.

Mail Online reported that men who have been cursed with a less-than-generous handout in the pants department might want to look away. New research published in September 2012 by the *Journal of Sexual Medicine* had shown that contrary to some popular (wishful?) thinking, penis size does matter when it comes to pleasing a woman in bed. The report stated that women who have frequent vaginal orgasms are more likely than other women to say they climax more easily with men with larger penises.

MICROPENIS: The Long and Short of It

Stuart Brody, the psychologist at the University of the West of Scotland who conducted the research, asked a sample of 323 women about their previous sexual encounters. They were asked whether penis length influenced their abilities to orgasm with vaginal stimulation.

Defining 'average' as the length of a twenty-pound note, which is 5.8 inches (or 14.9 centimetres), researchers asked women if they were more likely to orgasm vaginally with a longer-than-average or shorter-than-average penis.

Supporting the hypothesis that size matters, Brody and his colleagues found the women who reported the highest number of vaginal orgasms in the past month were most likely to say that longer was better. Brody told *Live Science*, 'This might be due at least in part to greater ability of a longer penis to stimulate the entire length of the vagina and the cervix.'

Now onto a less-scientific approach, in my first book I reported about a dating agency called the Hung Jury, based in the United States. There is a more-recent dating agency available for women who are looking for suitable well-endowed men. Call them Size Queens if you must, but the bottom line is that they do like their partners to have a big penis.

The dating agency is available to people online, and it's called 7orbetter.com. The introduction goes as follows: 'Welcome to 7orBetter. com, the well-endowed dating site and personal service that gives you what you really want. And what do you really want? Looks, humour, and intelligence are just an example of what initially draws us to another person. But if we are really truthful, there are other reasons. We are all attracted and drawn to size. The most common examples of greater size would be in reference to a woman's breasts or a man's manhood. This dating site is dedicated to quality singles who appreciate quality well-endowed men.'

Under the heading 'Dating Testimonials', the following comments, statements, and opinions are listed:

Size Queens

'I don't know where to begin. This site is *pure* genius! Yes I want a quality man, and yes, size does matter to me. I met my quality man on this site, and I was not disappointed later on. Thank you, 7orbetter.com!'

'Yes, size does matter to me, and there is no comparison when it comes to being with a man who is large. I like this site in particular because it is not just about the sexual aspect. It is seriously about dating and meeting great people.'

'Not sure if this will be posted or not because I am still looking for Mr Right. But at least I know that I can find Mr Right and that he will have what it takes to please me! I'm so glad that this is a respectable site that has no nudity. I'm very comfortable to be on here and not embarrassed who knows.'

'Hee hee…Well, um, OK…Size does matter, and it's not shallow to say so. It saves embarrassment should there be intimacy.'

'Well, I can only answer for myself. Yes, size matters a great deal. It is completely different being with a man who is five inches than being with a man who is nine inches. Yes, for some reason, there is a social stigma attached to women wanting a better-equipped man. I would be interested to hear why other people think this is so. For me, I can't help thinking it is a sort of conspiracy of men who are average or small.'

'I am a shy girl. I want to meet a quality guy, and I hate to admit this, but the guy needs to be big. This is a respectable site, no naked pictures, and I am not embarrassed to be here. I can find someone nice and know he is big enough for me. This site is *perfect* for me. Thank you to the creators for having the insight to build this site!'

Well, there you are, just ordinary women expressing their preferences for a man who has a larger penis. If you read the above testimonials carefully, you will see that they want well-endowed men who aren't complete knuckleheads, without any feelings towards their female partners. Furthermore, I should think *all* the women belonging to this dating agency do not want boring, lazy, foul-smelling men who think women are only good for one thing.

MICROPENIS: The Long and Short of It

The only men frightened, if that's the right word, of this dating agency are those who are full of their own self-importance and who have small penises. Apparently, some of the men who belong to the group of males who suffer from micropenis or from small penis syndrome over-compensate by being big-headed. This is sad, but unfortunately true.

Now I must inform you about a dating agency that leave you requiring a stay in intensive care. The agency is called Size Minded, and boy, is it!

Size Minded is owned by two well-endowed straight guys from Melbourne, Australia, and a small group of volunteers. The site grew out of frustrations with existing dating sites, which completely avoid the issue of penis size. The owners state that they are not associated with any other sites. They go on to say that they value their members' privacy and that no personal details or pictures are shown without express permission.

Under the heading 'Well-Endowed Dating', it informs interested parties that it is a free dating agency for well-endowed men and those who seek them. The men have to specify the length and girth of their penises and are allowed to upload explicit pictures to their galleries. Any users are able to specify the size ranges they are looking for and search the size/location to find their size match.

Here I must warn you to avert your eyes until the next paragraph unless you're happy to read some fruity language along with some eye-watering statistics. Under the headline 'Big Cocks, Huge Dicks, Massive Members', the following sentence appears: 'Our well-endowed men have penis sizes anywhere from a bit bigger than average to well over twelve inches and thicker than your wrist! You are more than welcome to have a look at some of these super-sized men if you are aged eighteen or over.' I will make the observation that if Long Dong Silver's penis (eighteen inches)—mentioned in my previous book—was a fake, there's no doubting the authentic penis on show from an unnamed member of this site. Truly, on the sight of this prize-winning penis, hanging down to its owner's knees, will make women sigh and men cry.

Next we have this confirmation verification service: 'All profiles are real. We don't tolerate fakers and remove them from the site. In addition, we offer a free gender and size verification service so you can be sure that what you see is what you get.'

If you want, and it's only if you want, you can see these things with your own eyes on the website. The males will list their ages, heights, eye colours, hair colours, lifestyles—such as smoker or drinker—whether they have any children, if they are married, and what their employment statuses are. Of course, there's the small matter of size, or rather, the large matter of size. The male will verify his penis length and girth when aroused. If a woman wants to see a man's penis when excited she can do so.

The women also state all the same details as above, such as ages, heights, eye colours, etc. They will also stipulate their preferences in terms of size. For example, one woman, aged thirty-three, wanted to meet a man 'between ten and thirteen inches in length.' She also wanted a penis measuring 'between six and eight inches in girth.'

I'm not saying that, if I were lucky enough to be this magnificently endowed, I would join this particular dating agency, but it would be very reassuring to know I could if I so desired.

To add to list of such dating sites, there's one simply called 'The Well-Hung Club'. If you are a woman and you're interested in looking at the men on display, don't let me delay you!

For a bit of humour you can always look up the 'Happy Pecker' website (apologies if I've mention this one before—I don't think I have, but there're so many of them!). It is the usual suspects, most of them, and they are all enormously endowed. It's all been done in the best possible taste, and if you believe that you'd believe anything!

I still have occasional nightmares about Margi Clarke as she appeared in *The Good Sex Guide*, walking through the communal showers while several men were lathering themselves up. I can still hear the spaghetti western music in the background while Ms Clarke dries her forehead with a towel after seeing all those naked men in the shower room. Flaccid penises appeared on the TV screen with their erect measurements beside the photographs. My God, how I suffered huge dollops of envy and feelings of inadequacy.

The knockout blow was in the following series, *The Good Sex Guide Abroad,* when Margi explained, 'I don't measure them [penises] myself; I weigh them!' To this, David Brian would say to Margi, if she encountered some of the men belonging to the Size Minded agency she better have some bloody big scales to weigh them!

CHAPTER SEVEN

You Just Wouldn't Believe It

Some things you read or hear about do seem to defy belief. Please consider this following scenario.

The headline that caught my eye is this one: 'Woman Divorces Her Husband because He Has a Five-Centimetre Penis'. The story unfolds as follows, 'The news that a woman, known only as Zhang, fifty-two, split with her other half, Zhou, because she was unhappy with the size of his manhood will do little to dampen the inadequate feeling many men already have about that part of their bodies.'

We find out that the then newly divorced woman from Taiwan had even gone a step further and actually detailed the size of the man's private parts, according to the *Daily Chilli*. Zhang explained, 'His penis is so small. It's like a kid's—only five centimetres long.' She also said, 'We've never had sex in our entire marriage.'

The two met in July 2008 and got married five months later. Zhang wanted to have sex prior to the ceremony, but he refused on religious grounds. She discovered the 'issue' on their wedding night, and she asked him to seek treatment.

However, they separated the day after, but had spent some nights together since then to see if the treatment had an effect. It hadn't. Who says that size doesn't matter? What was the treatment?

MICROPENIS: The Long and Short of It

To have only a five-centimetre (two-inch) penis can be traumatic—certainly for the man, but also for the female partner. Again, we must remember that one in two hundred men has an abnormally small penis. That's fact, not fiction.

Another eye-catching article was one with the headline 'Man Faces Divorce After Penis Extension Breaks During Sex'. The report went on, 'A man is being divorced by his wife after his penis extension broke off during sex. Doctors in Voronezh, southern Russia, had fitted the special prosthetic when Grigory Toporov, forty-seven, told them he didn't measure up to his wife's expectations in the bedroom. But she was horrified when the extension broke off during a passionate sex session.'

'I told her I would get a new one, but she wasn't having any of it. She said she was fed up with my failures in bed and wanted a divorce', said Toporov.

Another amazing story, to me at least, was news about a guy I had seen on the Internet under the title, 'Measuring up with "Unhung Hero" Patrick Moote'. The story read: 'The YouTube video of Patrick Moote having his marriage proposal rejected before a stadium full of people received ten million views in ten days. It was covered on major news stations and national talk shows. If this public humiliation wasn't emasculating enough, Moote's ex claimed one of the reasons she couldn't marry him was that his penis was too small.'

As a result Moote went on a globetrotting quest to answer two questions that are fundamental to masculine identity: 1. Does penis size really matter? and 2. Are there any safe methods for increasing your penis size? The 'cockumentary', as it's called, looks at his travels from porn conventions to encounters with 'dick doctors' in third-world motel rooms. Furthermore he discusses this subject with doctors, anthropologists, people who sell penis pumps, and so-called sexperts like Carol Queen, Dan Savage, and Annie Sprinkle.

He then gets the opinions of a few porn stars like Ron Jeremy, Andy San Dimas, Allie Haze, and Axel Braun, and chats with the man with the world's largest penis, Jonah Falcon.

Moote was then interviewed and asked why he chose to propose to his girlfriend in such a public way, during the UCLA basketball game. He replied that it seemed like a sweet idea at the time, although he admitted he's not sure why. Then he was asked how long it took him after the video went viral to decide to make a film of his 'problem'. Moote replied that it wasn't a publicity stunt, but he discussed it with one of his friends, Brian Spitz, and they decided to make a video on the question, 'does size matter?' After a few drinks together they decided to go ahead with the film.

The sixty-four-thousand-dollar question was, why wasn't his ex-girl-friend, who rejected his marriage proposal, interviewed? Moote admitted that he took things she had told him in private and made them everybody's business, which was really unfair. However, he said that although she wasn't 'in love with idea', she was cool with the idea.

He was also asked why he dwelt on the point that his other ex-girl-friends admitted he had a small penis instead of thinking, 'I may have a small penis, yet it hasn't stopped me from dating all these attractive women.' Moote's reply was simply that his charm outweighed his penis—in fact, most things outweighed his penis at that point.

The interviewer then asked him why the 'enhanced' penises of men who underwent penile surgery were never shown on film. The reply from Moote was that the surgery definitely works—'it adds a bunch of girth'—but the problem was getting them on camera. Moote said he could understand this, since if they were insecure enough to have penis enlargement surgery, having it filmed was probably their biggest nightmare.

On the Internet there's a comment by an individual that this subject matter of the micropenis had already been done. The message board continued, 'The TV documentary was called *Me, My Penis, and I*. The man's partner really didn't care and truly loved him, but he was still bothered by it. It really [is] a case of, if the woman loves you she won't care what size you are.'

Now, let me say in my own voice that I don't believe that's true. Women can fall in love with whomever they like—perhaps a serial killer or a smelly man with bad breath—but that fact hardly gives a man comfort. For the record, the actual title was just *My Penis and I*. If you've read page eighty of my previous book, you will know that our old friend Lawrence Barraclough's girlfriend, Nicola, when asked by Mr Barraclough himself if she wished he had a bigger penis, replied, 'I do, yes.' Sometimes I feel like pulling my hair out!

There's one story about one man's incident that I did not mention at all in my first book. To me it would have needed another chapter, or even another book, to discuss this incredible story. This happened twenty years ago…

A man named John Wayne Bobbitt hit the world headlines when his then-wife, Lorena, chopped off his penis with an eight-inch kitchen knife. Newspapers like the *Sun* tell us that men all over the world wince when they hear about the attack on Mr Bobbitt's manhood.

However, on June 24, 2013, a story in the *Sun* was headlined with 'My wife did me a favour, chopping off my willy…I've slept with seventy girls since.' The paper then followed with these statistics: one hundred forty-one—the number of reported cases of a lover cutting off a man's penis; ten hours—the length of the operation to reattach Bobbitt's penis; twelve weeks—the amount of time before Bobbitt had sex again; and three—the number of times he has been married.

Bobbitt did admit to the reporter that people thought it was all a big joke but that he almost bled to death. He explained, 'After the knife sliced through, I lost a huge amount of blood.' At some point he passed out, and when he came round, he was being prepared for surgery.

You Just Wouldn't Believe It

His wife had sliced off the top two and a half inches, and the doctors had to reattach all the nerve endings and tissue. The procedure was obviously a very delicate operation. Bobbitt woke up to find that he was covered in bandages and that they had inserted a catheter tube—and for two months, that was the only way he could go to the bathroom.

The doctors explained there could be all sorts of complications. The worst-case scenario was if an infection set in to such an extent his penis would go black and drop off.

Bobbitt's notoriety began the night he stumbled back to his Virginia home following an evening's drinking and started arguing with his wife. It was June 23, 1993.

His wife claimed he raped her that night, but he was acquitted of this when the case went to court. According to Bobbitt, he was asleep when she went downstairs, grabbed an eight-inch kitchen knife, and attacked him. She then drove off, hurling his severed penis into a nearby field, before realising what she had done and calling the emergency services. Bobbitt was taken to hospital and, after a painstaking search by emergency teams, the missing part was found and put on ice, ready to be reattached.

Lorena said in court that her husband had been sexually, physically, and emotionally abusive during their four-year marriage, and she was found not guilty of malicious wounding on the grounds of temporary insanity.

Three months afterwards, he met a woman in a bar who obviously recognised him from all the media attention. Then, to quote Bobbitt, 'We went back to her place and did what comes naturally. I was frightened it wouldn't work, and my penis wasn't 100 percent, but we did OK.'

He told the reporter that it took two years to fully heal, and once it did, he set about making full use of it. Although some doctors told him he would never be able to have sex again, because his injuries were so bad, Bobbitt proved them wrong, and he's slept with seventy women since the incident.

MICROPENIS: The Long and Short of It

John Bobbitt became a global celebrity—with television and radio shows queueing up to interview him. The *Howard Stern Show* offered to pay for a penis enlargement, and Bobbitt jumped at the chance. Bobbitt explained that he had not fully regained his confidence in that department, and he wanted the operation to help him get back his self-esteem. Newspaper readers then discovered that the penis-enlargement operation added nearly two inches to the length of his penis. He also had his girth increased.

That was when Bobbitt soon began to take advantage of his notoriety by forming a band called the Severed Parts when he moved to Las Vegas. While there, he made a couple of adult films, including one called *Frankenpenis*.

Regarding his personal life, however, he found himself on a dark path. In 1994 Bobbitt was jailed for fifteen days for beating his fiancée, Kristina Elliott. There was no wedding. His wedding in 2001 to a businesswoman lasted just twenty-three days. Then there was a third marriage in 2002, which lasted two years, during which time he was arrested for assaulting his wife.

Apparently he has now given up his hard-living days, and the violent attacks are things of the past. He has found God and moved back to New York, where he plans to settle down with a woman who has known him since childhood.

Before too long he will release his autobiography. I will bet any money you'd like that he doesn't have to self-publish his own book like yours truly. I'm certainly not bitter; it's just a statement of fact.

What have I got in common with Bobbitt? In many ways nothing at all—I've never been to jail, and I've certainly never been to bed with seventy women. I would also have to say that I've never had my penis cut off, and I hope I never do! And I've never beaten anyone up, woman or man.

However there are a few things, I suppose. Yes, I've had my penis surgically enhanced for a number of reasons, one of which was to increase my self-esteem. Added to which I've been on television documentaries (mind you, Bobbitt has probably been on more talk shows than I've had hot dinners), and I've been on a radio programme. These things you'll know by reading my first book. If you haven't read it yet, don't hesitate to order it. I just know you'll buy a copy of Mr Bobbitt's book, but my book is cheaper, and I would like to think it's every bit as good.

Speaking of the *Howard Stern Show,* I saw something on the Internet that left me open-mouthed. How these guys had the courage to appear on his show I simply do not know. There was a filmed section of Mr Stern's show, which had the title 'The Smallest Penis Contest', and I simply cannot understand how most of these guys had the courage, or shall I say balls, to appear on screen. Their 'job' was to stand in single file until they were asked to step forward to a studio technician with a microphone—all this while they were completely naked!

The head of the proceedings was Howard Stern himself, with his microphone and headphones on, introducing the contestants one by one. Then there were four panellists judging these poor men as they stepped up to the plate.

The first man, although the panel and Stern thought he looked more like a woman, who like me, before my operation, had nothing 'down there', spoke about his problem. The one woman on the panel, named Robin, couldn't stop laughing, spluttering, 'He doesn't have one!' Then she made the observation that the guy needed a breast reduction and a penis enlargement. Which was very near the knuckle, but in all honesty, it was true. Robin couldn't believe her eyes and asked the poor man, 'Do you actually have sex?' Before this guy went off camera, the panel all agreed he had no penis to see, and he had, at least, C-cup breasts. All this can be looked up on the Internet.

Each guy stepped forward and answered questions about his tiny penis. Howard Stern admitted that 'it takes a lot of guts' to do what they were putting themselves through.

MICROPENIS: The Long and Short of It

I must admit I didn't watch the whole video—it just reminded me of how tiny I was and all the awful problems it gave me. Maybe it did make me feel a bit better about myself, seeing guys as small as I had been before 1996, but overall it just made me feel sorry for the poor men involved.

Meanwhile, there's the other extreme. There's always the other extreme. In *Cosmopolitan,* an article written by Natasha Burton listed eleven famous penises, or at least, men with famous penises.

Number one was Rasputin, who apparently possessed a penis measuring eleven inches when only *flaccid*! His member rests in a jar at a Russian erotica museum. I don't travel myself, but it would be interesting to hear from any readers who have seen this for real.

Number two was Casanova, who was listed on the basis that his penis was always busy because he had reputedly bedded many women.

Number three was Michelangelo's statue of David, which is acknowledged as the most famous statue in history. Please see my book cover!

Number four was John Holmes, who was a prolific porn star, who reportedly had a fourteen-inch, or perhaps thirteen and a half inch penis. I would like to be so worried to argue about half an inch. Before my first operation in 1996, I only had a one inch when soft (half an inch when cold).

Number five was Ron Jeremy, a porn star with a penis measuring nine-and-three-quarters inches.

Number six was Wilt Chamberlain, who is an NBA legend, and who has been said to have bedded over twenty-four thousand women. How he ever got time to play any basketball is a question that needs to be asked.

Number seven is the late Errol Flynn, who once played 'You Are My Sunshine' on piano with his very large penis at a party. Talk about a show-off!

You Just Wouldn't Believe It

Number eight is Tommy Lee, who was filmed having sex with his then-wife Pamela Anderson, and apparently it left no doubt that he is very large down below.

Number nine is the aforementioned John Wayne Bobbitt. Nothing else needs to be said.

Number ten is Jon Hamm, who is an actor and renowned for his extremely large manhood.

Number eleven is none other than Jonah Falcon, who currently claims the record for the largest penis in the world—thirteen and a half inches—and being interviewed on daytime television, if you please. He may not have been seen naked, but I can imagine thousands, if not millions, of men feeling incredibly inadequate when hearing about his vital statistics.

If you want to actually see incredibly large men—as opposed to just reading about them—you can view any of the hundreds, or even thousands, of websites showing these men in all their glory. There's one called 'Famous Big Peckers', which sounds humorous, at least until you see the subheading 'Take a gander and see how you measure up to some of the world's longest cocks.' My self-esteem takes a dive when I actually see the likes of Ron Jeremy, Richard Mann (eleven inches), Fredrick Lamont (known as Mandingo, eleven and a half), the late John Holmes, and, of course, Jonah Falcon.

What to see? *The Smallest Penis Contest* or 'The Famous Big Peckers'; you pay your money and you take your choice. If you see the first, you might feel really proud of your manhood or, unless you're very fortunate, you might see the second and feel extremely inadequate.

CHAPTER EIGHT

A Funny Thing Happened At the Welbeck Clinic on October 5, 2011

I had made an appointment to see my surgeon, Dr Gary Horn, at the Welbeck Hospital, 27 Welbeck Street in London on Wednesday, October 5, 2011. I intended to ask him if he could get rid of a large deposit of fat that had collected over my left eyelid. The fat had gradually built up over a number of years and was apparently due to my high cholesterol. Although it didn't require any medication, I was advised by my GP to keep a sensible diet. When I asked him if he could do anything about the actual collection of fat, he just shrugged his shoulders and replied, 'Well I can't, because it's cosmetic.'

The other reason I wanted to see Dr Horn was to check on the two penoplasty procedures where he enhanced the girth of my penis. I was very happy with the results of the two procedures, but I just wanted to have his reassurance.

My appointment was for 10:00 a.m., and I had to make a reasonably early start from home to catch the appropriate train to get there in good time. I made the journey in good time and reported to the reception, where a young gentleman welcomed me. He was extremely helpful and told me to take a seat, and then he was good enough to bring me a lovely, refreshing cup of tea.

A Funny Thing Happened At the Welbeck Clinic ...

I sat there reading my newspaper and passing the time of day with the young man. He informed me that he had to be on reception for at least twelve hours a day, less his lunch hour. I really was impressed with his whole demeanour and efficiency.

When I had been waiting for over half an hour, he volunteered to contact Dr Horn to see how much longer I would have to wait before his arrival at the clinic. I was told perhaps another hour. I thanked him for finding out this information.

Dr Horn had to travel to the United Kingdom from Paris, so I wasn't particularly surprised he was running late. The receptionist was good enough to make me another cup of tea—this time with biscuits. I continued to read my paper.

A few other clients had arrived by now to see various other surgeons who performed surgery at the Welbeck Hospital. I noticed a couple of women and another man who had his head stuck in a newspaper, trying no doubt to look uninterested in other patients.

At this point a woman in her mid- to late forties (I would guess) sat next to me. What happened over the next ten or so minutes left me gobsmacked. She started talking to me as though she had known me for years. Anyone watching would have thought we were best buddies.

She made no secret of the fact that she had undergone a breast enlargement. How can I put this? She had on a very low-cut top and displayed a very large cleavage. I did my best not to notice—honest, readers, I really did. I felt myself blushing just as if I was in my teens.

She informed me her surgeon was French and that he was a fantastic surgeon. Her next sentence floored me, because she said that she would have no hesitation in recommending him to my wife! I wanted to say to her, 'Steady on, love, we've only been talking for a couple of minutes; anyway you've never met her.'

The lady then started telling me about her eighteen-year-old daughter, who had already undergone a breast enlargement. She proceeded to show me some photos on her mobile phone of her daughter in a bikini—some photos were before her operation and some after the operation. Mightily impressive, but I didn't really need or want to see these photographs.

She informed me that her daughter wanted to be a glamour model. Apparently, she was going to support her daughter all she could so that her daughter's dreams would come true.

She also told me she had a son aged thirteen, who she said was going to be very handsome one day, even though he wasn't what she called 'photogenic' at that time. She also had an eight-year-old daughter, who, according to her, was definitely photogenic. I felt I was being swept away by a tidal wave, and I had no strength to stop it.

She then asked me who my surgeon was, after I had mentioned my surgeon was French as well. When she discovered my surgeon was Dr Horn, a huge smile appeared on her face. She leaned forward and, somewhat more quietly, informed me her husband had also had a procedure done by Dr Horn. In a hushed tone, she informed me that her husband had undergone penis-enlargement surgery.

Then, still in a hushed tone, she asked me the sixty-four-thousand-dollar question, 'What procedure did you have?' I felt my face go beetroot red as I whispered, 'I had penis enlargement as well.' She obviously saw and sensed my embarrassment, and almost in a motherly way replied, 'It's nothing to be ashamed about. My husband and I are very happy with the results—are you happy with yours?' I replied that I was. She said with a knowing sort of smile, 'Look, love, thousands of men have had it done. I do think it seems embarrassing for men to admit having that done, but really they shouldn't be embarrassed.'

During this discussion between us, if that's what it was, more people had arrived to sit in the waiting area. My new friend then noticed two women on the other side of the room. They looked liked mother and daughter and, sure enough, they were. Without a hint of embarrassment, the lady next to me said to the mother, 'You look gorgeous. My God, you look as young as your daughter.' The mother looked across with a great big smile and said, 'Thanks for the compliment.'

A Funny Thing Happened At the Welbeck Clinic ...

My friend said, 'God knows what she's having done. She doesn't look as though she needs anything done.' I wondered what the woman was going to say next. But then salvation appeared as Dr Horn arrived with his suitcase direct from his journey to St. Pancras. He nodded and asked me to follow him into his consulting room. Escape at last!

When I sat down in his room, I asked Dr Horn if he could perform the minor procedure of taking away the fatty deposit from over my left eyelid. He examined it and said that he could perform that procedure with a local anaesthetic and a prescription of eye drops.

Then I asked him about the last two penile girth enhancements he had performed for me. He examined me and confirmed that the fat transfer would last as long as I do. My girth would remain and no fat would be reabsorbed from my penis into my body. I was extremely happy at this news.

Dr Horn let me use his top-of-the-line camera to take his photograph for my book *Penoplasty: A True Story*.

I shook his hand, wished him well, and said I would see him sometime in the near future. I walked out of the room into the reception area looking straight ahead in case I met up with my new friend. What a day, what a woman, but most of all, what wonderful news about my girth!

Since my visit to the Welbeck Hospital in 2011, I can inform you that I returned there on March 19, 2014, and this time it was a bit more relaxed, as I didn't have that brazen, but very nice, lady there to flaunt her cleavage and to ask me who my surgeon was. I was looked after by another very pleasant young man at the reception desk. He informed me that the previous young man on the desk had left to become a nurse.

About half an hour after my arrival I met Anna Camilleri, who showed me the few paragraphs she had put together for this book. As you would have seen from her comments, she knows what she is talking about, having spent over twelve years as a consultant in the field of cosmetic surgery. We than went over to a plush hotel lobby to have a wonderfully refreshing nonalcoholic cocktail drink, with coffee to follow, as we continued our conversation about my book. She generously paid for the refreshments, and I promised I would return the compliment on my next visit.

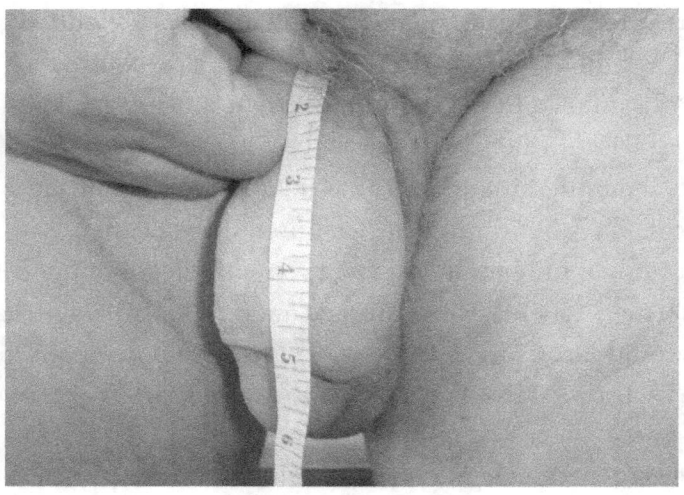

6 inch flaccid length after penoplasty

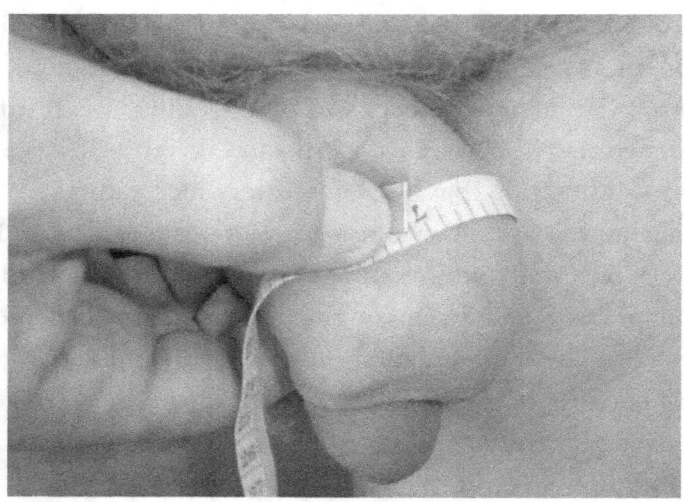

7inch flaccid girth after penoplasty

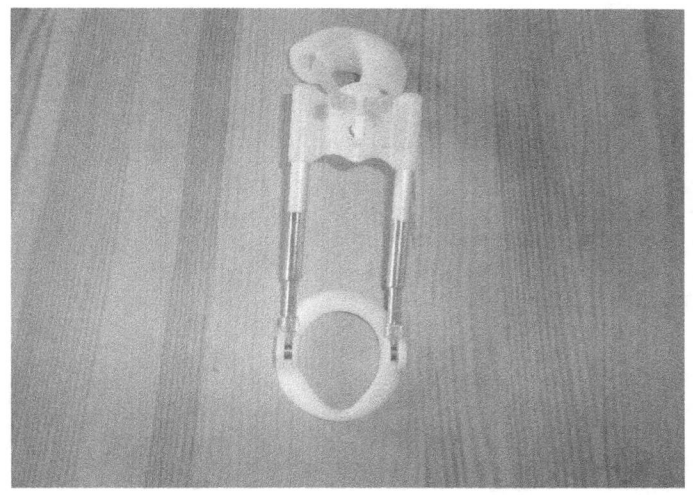

Andro Penis or JES Extender

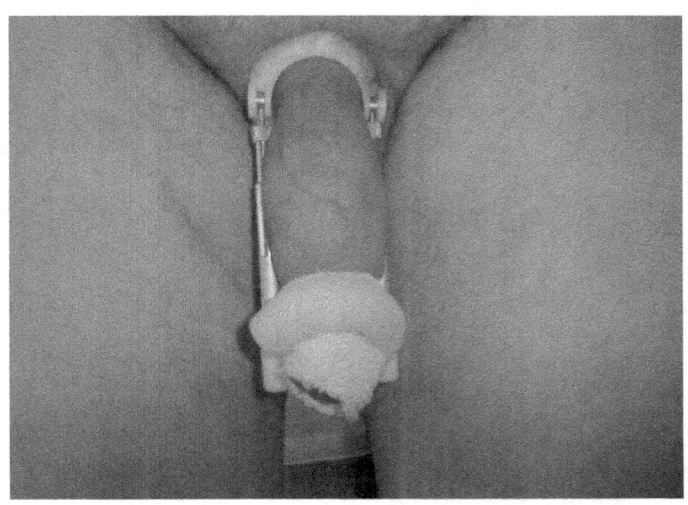

Andro Penis being worn after penoplasty

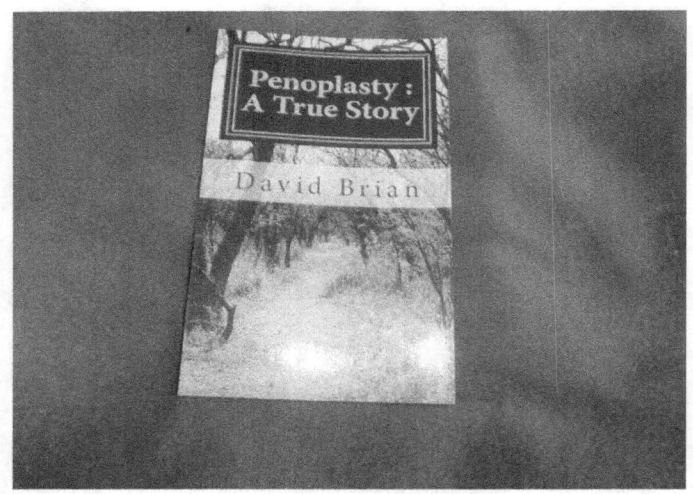

My first book Penoplasty: A True Story

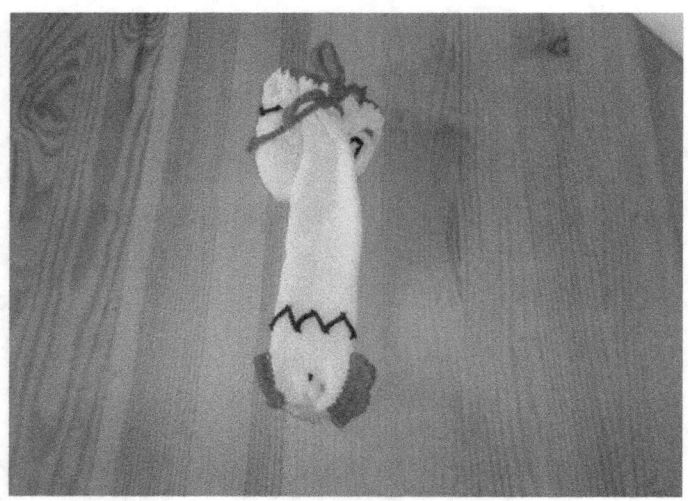

Willy Warmer

CHAPTER NINE

Penis Management

I was reading a page of the *Guardian* on August 8, 2013, when I came across a piece by Suzanne Moore on 'good penis management'. Interesting, I thought to myself as I started reading the piece while having my cup of morning char.

Her article started like this, 'In light of the "cock au vin" story, here is my guide to what not to do with your penis.'

1. Do not involve your penis in sexting if you are [a] public figure with a penchant for extramarital affairs. Pictures of the engorged members of members of Parliament will leak. As Anthony Weiner found, sexting is best left to teenagers, who at least know what Snapchat is. Why say it with flowers when you can say it with a shot of your erection under the desk? Romance is not dead.

2. Do not neglect your penis. I am talking hygiene. Women are subjected to pharmacy aisles full of fresheners, wipes, and sprays that encourage us to believe that without them our genital area is just a smelly, slimy mess, but there is no equivalent for men. Surely there is a gap in the market for products to encourage men to stay box fresh under their boxers.

3. Do not stick your penis into household objects, however tempting. Since the fire brigade has had to warn men not to put their

genitals in toasters, we are reminded of all the A&E stories of the many men who get their tackle trapped in everything from radiators to vacuum cleaners.

4. Do not use your penis to urinate all over the place in public. Why on earth is this acceptable? I am no prude, but often when I am walking home, I see guys staggering about peeing randomly into gardens, bus stops, and doorways. It is smelly, horrible, and antisocial.

5. Do not ever put your penis into someone who does not want this. Even if the person is drunk. Or if you two are married. This is rape. There is never any excuse. Ever.

6. Do not name your penis. Poor Justin Bieber's has been named 'Jerry' by his fans. Message boards are full of young women and men with naming problems. 'My boyfriend wants me to call his penis Cockosaurus Rex', for example. Who am I to say otherwise? Well, I am me, and I say otherwise.

7. Do not derive pleasure from your penis with other men. In thirty-eight African countries homosexuality is illegal. The situation in Russia is dire, with Vladimir Putin pushing forward antigay legislation and neo-Nazis beating and even killing gay people. This is why Stephen Fry is rightly calling for Russia to be stripped of the Winter Olympics. (Regrettably they weren't.)

8. Do not pierce your own penis. All I am saying is, do what thou wilt to you manhood, but safely. Piercing risks HIV and hepatitis B and C if not done properly.

9. Do not try to make your penis bigger by buying Bazooka Pills or other rubbish offered online. Penile implants can wreck lives. Lengthening surgery, if you really want to know, means 'severing the suspensory ligament that holds the penile shaft inside the body'. Girth can be added by attaching tissue sheets of AlloDerm. What is AlloDerm? 'It is cadaver skin that has had its cells removed, leaving simply collagen.' Nice.

Penis Management

10. Do not mistake your penis for your brain. The silly idea that men possess wicked willies and can't help acting on impulse is surely rather insulting?

After reading the article I took it upon myself to write a response to Ms Moore addressing all of her ten penis-management points. Along with my letter I enclosed a copy of my first book *Penoplasty: A True Story*, so she could see I knew a thing or two about some of the details she mentioned in her article.

Regarding point one, I stated categorically to her that I've certainly never done this thing called 'sexting' of one's penis. In fact I've never even sent a text to any person. Believe it or not! Why any man would send a photo of his penis to an unknown person—man or woman—is beyond me. Would it be done to shock them? Would it be to repulse them? Would it be to impress them? To me this sounds very similar to a pathetic little man flashing his penis at a woman. This is a total no-no, and surely every right-minded person knows that.

Having seen certain TV programmes on channel four about teenage schoolchildren, I learned that they can and they do send each other parts of their anatomy via these damned mobiles and other machines I don't even know the names of.

Point two concerns Suzanne's request that men keep themselves fresh and scrupulously clean. I don't know any excuse for men not being clean unless they are living out on the streets. The points made by Ms Moore are totally kosher, and they do not need any further comments. I'm left wondering if Suzanne has had some rather unfortunate encounters with some dubious men.

In point three Ms Moore asks men not to stick their penises into household objects for sexual pleasure! Presumably there have been some extremely embarrassing events where men have to be taken to the nearest A&E to rescue their penises from a vacuum cleaner.

MICROPENIS: The Long and Short of It

Honestly, I've heard it all now. In all my time on this planet, I've never ever wanted to place my manhood into a toaster or some other home appliance. It's never been big enough to do such a thing, but even if it were bigger, I cannot for the life of me think about why a man wants to do such a stupid thing. I informed Suzanne Moore of this in no uncertain terms.

Next we have point four, where Ms Moore has personally witnessed men urinating in public, without a care in the world. She informs *Guardian* readers that it is antisocial and castigates men stupid enough to do such childish things. Alcohol does things to people of both sexes, and I've often felt sorry for the street cleaners who have the job of hosing down streets and shop doorways first thing in the morning. I can't say I don't agree with her on this point as well. I do not drink alcohol at all, but even if I did have the odd pint, I certainly wouldn't go round peeing all over the place.

Point five brings up the problem with men who want to put their penis into women, men, or any other living creatures who do not want this process to take place. Again, I'm in total agreement with Ms Moore. Men please take note of this.

Well, I was waiting for this one to come along. Number six finds Suzanne saying she doesn't like it when a man (or presumably also a woman) calls the male phallus by a silly name. The example she gave—'Cockosaurus Rex'—is indeed something to make you wince with embarrassment, I quite agree. But she does refer to consenting adults, and I think it's a case of what makes you and your partner happy. That means you can go ahead and call your bits anything you like. What consenting couples do in the privacy of their bedroom is nothing to do with me, or indeed Ms Moore.

Point seven brings an extremely serious point concerning men who derive pleasure from their penises together with other men. Ms Moore mentions the appalling situation in a number of countries where homosexuality is illegal. It makes you wonder how backward we still are when people are not allowed to be open about their sexuality.

Point eight, I must admit, brought tears to my eyes. Suzanne pleaded for men not to pierce their own penises. All I can say is that I totally concur with her again. She brings attention to the fact that when not done properly, self-piercing can give an unfortunate man HIV or hepatitis B and C. I've had my penis enlarged surgically because I absolutely needed it, as it was classed as a micropenis. Men who pierce their manhood are doing it presumably for decoration. I wouldn't do that in a million years, but for men who want it done, go to a place that specialises in that sort of thing!

Now we get to my area of expertise in point nine. Suzanne Moore tells men not to buy Bazooka pills or any other rubbish that's offered online, and as far as I'm concerned I'm in total agreement. Then we're told that penile implants can wreck lives. To that I say that crossing the road can wreck a person's life, if you're knocked over by a lorry. I haven't had an implant and I'll bet Ms Moore hasn't either. Looking up 'What is the success rate for penile implants?' on the relevant page of a surgeon's book, we discover the facts shown below.

'Regardless of the model chosen, patients and their partners report a high overall degree of satisfaction with penile implants (also called penile prosthesis). Of 425 men in a British study of penile implants, most of whom had the malleable variety, 89 percent could have sexual intercourse, and 81 percent were satisfied with the implant results'. Implants are primarily for men who have erectile dysfunction.

Lengthening surgery, which I've had, proved to be very effective. As I have had this process and Ms Moore has not, I feel comfortable contradicting her. She states correctly that the major surgical procedure is to cut the suspensory ligament. When performed properly this does increase the length between one to two inches. By using the JES Extender, Andropenis, or the plain simple penis stretcher, further gains of between one to two inches can be achieved. When I told Glyn Drewe at the Belvedere Clinic that my wife was expecting a baby, she rather cheekily replied, 'See, it still works.' The surgery, if done correctly, will not impair a man's sexual functioning. I'm living proof of that.

Girth, we are told by Ms Moore, can be added by attaching AlloDerm. She describes AlloDerm as 'cadaver skin that has had its cells removed, leaving simply collagen'. Her final word is 'nice'. As we all should know, sarcasm is the lowest form of wit. For Suzanne's information, AlloDerm has been used to repair hernias and in breast-reconstruction postmastectomy procedures. It's also been introduced for use in dentistry and the treatment and repair of burns. Like every surgical procedure, it has to be used correctly, and after-care is also very important. However, from my research, it has produced excellent results for penile girth enhancement.

My girth increases have been produced by harvesting fat from my inner thighs (my first three operations), and my last operation harvested fat from my buttocks, which was done by Dr Gary Horn. The first procedure (1996) did leave two 'bumps' along the shaft of my penis. After my 'revision', my penis was much thicker than my original tiny size. My last two procedures, undertaken by Dr Horn, produced excellent results and *no* bruising—please take my word for it. Obviously I have never had AlloDerm to enlarge my girth, but from my research, it appears to give excellent results nine times out of ten. Please note however that no operation is guaranteed to be 100 percent successful.

It's a shame that such an intelligent person as Suzanne Moore ends up appearing to seem, on some subjects, not to know her arse from her elbow.

Her last point, number ten, tells gentlemen not to mistake their penises for their brains. Some men, how many we don't know, have wicked willies that can't stop acting on impulse. Do women have penis envy? Not as far as I'm aware—what the majority of women have is a preference regarding its size. Here endeth the tenth lesson.

I did say to Suzanne Moore that she has my permission to quote from my first book, and if I don't hear from her, I take it I can quote wholesale from her article. That's why, dear reader, you have been reading this chapter called 'Penis Management'.

CHAPTER TEN

Loose Women

There's a television programme on ITV, which has been on British TV screens since 1999 and has attracted lunchtime viewing figures of around a million or more people—*Loose Women*. My previous book described some of the topics covered by the all-female panel—penis size being one of them.

To be honest, I haven't seen it for a year or two, because some of the subject matter is painful to a man like me. Since I first saw the programme, a number of its panel have jumped ship, either voluntarily, or by orders of the management. Apparently the viewing figures as I write this chapter (March 2014) are spiralling down—perhaps because the most outspoken women on the panel, such as Carol McGiffen and Denise Welch, have gone on to pastures new.

One of the above-mentioned panellists no longer on the show is that shy, retiring actress named Denise Welch. One thing I have in common with Ms Welch is depression. She has spoken and written about this problem for a great number of years. I haven't, but I can admit I do suffer quite badly from depression, and I've been on medication for the last ten years.

Some of the depression goes back years, to when I was at school and had to suffer the sheer embarrassment of being in the showers after having PE. Having an almost nonexistent penis is the absolute pits.

Loose Women

It's enough to make any man depressed. Make no mistake, I felt so low sometimes, it really is difficult to find the words that can describe it.

Getting back to Denise Welch, the public discovered in the *Daily Mirror* on September 5, 2012, that she and Carol Vorderman exchanged saucy notes about men who were appearing on *Loose Women* either as guests or in the audience. Ms Welch revealed that they had great fun and would send each other little messages during the show, such as, 'How big do you think his willy is?' They would then draw diagrams of what size they thought it would be! Thank the Lord I never appeared on the show.

On March 14, 2013, Denise was interviewed by Jane Atkinson in the *Sun*. Along with the article, there was a photograph of her with her arms around her husband-to-be, Lincoln Townley. There were also several smaller photos with speech bubbles, indicating Ms Welch's views on a number of subjects.

One opinion concerned her boyfriend, Lincoln. 'We have passion in and out of the bedroom. We have a wonderful sex life.' No wonder she had a smile from ear to ear. Lucky lady or what? She has a man fourteen years her junior and plenty of fulfilment as well.

This article, however, gave me time to reflect on Jane Atkinson, as she was photographed with Denise Welch. It's true that it helps when you can put a face to a name. So this was the woman who phoned me on April 12, 2006, wanting me to be interviewed so that it would give hope to men who were poorly endowed like me. On page 165 of *Penoplasty: A True Story* I describe in detail how things panned out.

She had got my name and telephone number from an agency that I had signed up with. Ms Atkinson gave me the hard sell and insisted she could go ahead with my story, even if I didn't agree with her article. Furthermore she explained that she didn't like the way I was dressed in an article I gave for *Chat* magazine—I was wearing a T-shirt and jeans. She wanted me to be photographed in a suit for the article. I insisted that I would do an interview for the now-defunct *News of the World* Sunday paper, but I didn't want my photo to be included—suit or no suit.

MICROPENIS: The Long and Short of It

My previous book will outline how I felt I was being coerced into something I really didn't want to do. An article on penoplasty, which is, after all, a taboo subject, surely didn't require a photograph of me to validate the interview. 'Danny' on the *This Morning* TV show didn't have his face to the camera at all, and he was wearing a wig. We know that there were photos of his penis before and after the operation, but nevertheless his identity was protected. This didn't invalidate his story by any means.

I nevertheless still had several photographs taken by an agent of the *News of the World,* and he took photos of my letters from the Belvedere Private Clinic to prove I had actually undergone penile enlargement surgery. I felt like saying in my best cockney accent, 'Don't ya trust me, governor?'

What really got my goat was that on Good Friday in 2006, I had to go over to a local park in very heavy, drizzly rain to have a couple of dozen photographs taken for the newspaper. I even had to take my coat off and hang it on a wire fence—sometimes I really do despair.

Jane Atkinson was supposed to ring me at 10:30 a.m. the next day (a Saturday), but that call didn't materialise. Surprise, surprise. I had to phone her that afternoon to discover she would not run with the story in the next day's *News of the World*. She said that she didn't want to mess up my Easter holidays—she obviously realised I was concerned about having my photograph in the, best-selling Sunday newspaper in Britain. She said she would ring me on Tuesday, but unsurprisingly that call was never made, so I just breathed a huge sigh of relief.

I would have been happy to do the interview about my experiences of having a tiny penis and then having the enlargement surgery that has made such an improvement in my life. It would have been really good to put that message out to the one man in two hundred who suffers from an abnormally small penis. I've been advised not to mention money from the point of my being an interviewee, but I feel obliged to mention that Ms Atkinson did offer me a fair sum of money to undertake the interview. It was a fair sum, but it wasn't an eye-watering amount.

One more thing I would like to say about Jane Atkinson. In the *Guardian* newspaper on February 14, 2013, there was a piece under the

Loose Women

heading, 'Six ex-N o W Journalists Arrested in New Phone Hacking Inquiry.' One of the journalists arrested just happened to be 'the *Sun's* northern features editor, Jane Atkinson'.

All I will say on this subject is that whether Ms Atkinson is found innocent or guilty concerning phone hacking, I will not laugh or cry either way. I honestly feel that she did give me a bit of a hard time concerning the article, which was never published. A photograph can illustrate but words, honest words, I should stress, are the most important parts of an interview. My story was, and still remains, the truth. Sod the photograph of me in my Burton-manufactured England World Cup football suit— after all, what's that to do with me having a micropenis?

Apparently Carol McGiffin always fires straight from the hip, and during her ten years on *Loose Women* she's never been slow at coming forward. What's more, she wrote a book, but then who hasn't? It was published on May 27, 2010, and apparently tells the public, in a no-holds-barred manner, about her hard upbringing, which hasn't stopped her making a mark on society.

I haven't read her book, and maybe I never will, but I do remember some of the anecdotes she told on *Loose Women*. My cup of tea nearly finished on the other side of the dining room when she said she had had sex with about fifty guys! In a way, I respected her honesty and how she gave everybody this attitude, which seemed to say, 'I don't give a f**k what you think about me.' At that time she enjoyed being with blokes and obviously enjoyed sex. There's no way I would criticise her for that— if it had been a bloke bedding fifty women he would be called a stud.

She also mentioned on another occasion that she used to give her men marks out of ten in respect of their performances in bed. I don't think anybody will be surprised to learn Ms McGiffen would frighten the living daylights out of me. As I've reported before, when the *Loose Women* panel were discussing the *Sun's* 'Two Inch' article, about John Prescott, Carol laid it on the line by saying that she had a previous partner who 'was so small it was ridiculous'.

MICROPENIS: The Long and Short of It

From my own experience, this subject was discussed a number of times on the programme. Towards the end of my watching the programme, I do recall a panel, consisting of Carol, Denise Welch, Lisa Maxwell and one other who I can't remember. The first to answer the question, 'Is penis size important?' was Denise who stated categorically that penis size was important and informed us that when a penis is very small, a woman cannot feel it inside her vagina.

This opinion was totally agreed with by Carol, who said there was no other way of putting it—size was important. However, she mentioned a trip she and her boyfriend, Mark, took to the Far East, which was educational because there were some live sex shows where some of the men had 'massive ones' and even her other half felt a touch inadequate.

Lisa Maxwell agreed with the other women, saying she wouldn't want to be with a bloke so small that she would need to wear her glasses to see it! As I was once a tiny bloke myself, this is a 'real punch up the trousers'.

Lastly, Ms McGiffen mentioned numerous times that her boyfriend always wanted sex (go on, make me feel good about myself!) and that after coming out of the shower he invariably did his 'willy dance' to impress her. Whatever next, before you know it they'll be both appearing on *Strictly Come Dancing*!

I should point out that since I first had this book published (November 2014) Carol has been diagnosed with breast cancer. She is being treated for this disease and her boyfriend has been incredibly supportive. I wish her well – please God she overcomes this terrible disease.

Since this book was first published in November 2014 Carol McGiffen has been diagnosed with breast cancer. Her boyfriend has been more supportive than ever and I pray to God that she overcomes her illness.

CHAPTER ELEVEN

Micropenises

I vividly remember that some years ago, a very attractive woman said this about the male organ, 'With the increasing sexual objectification/pornification of women in our unequal society, it shouldn't be much of a surprise that the inadequacies of the male member still rarely gets publicly discussed—or, indeed, acknowledged that such inadequacies even exist.'

What I think the above statement shows is that, generally speaking, men have had it very cushy over the centuries, as it's always been women who have been judged on their looks and physical attributes, such as the size of their breasts. Even if it's a generalisation, at least it's been a very accurate and truthful one.

Last year I exchanged e-mails with a thoroughly pleasant, sensitive young man who had undergone penis-enlargement surgery by my surgeon Dr Gary Horn. He asked me for any information or tips regarding the stretcher commonly known as the JES Extender, the Andropenis, or, as it was called on the documentary *Drastic Plastic*, the penis stretcher.

The advice I gave the young man (I shall call him RP) was to take it step by step and not to rush things or to expect too much too soon. To make it less painful on his glans (commonly known as the helmet), he could use cotton wool or pieces of bandage.

MICROPENIS: The Long and Short of It

The last time I heard from RP, he was progressing nicely, and he felt happy with the increase in length. He did, however, have some fat reabsorbed, which lessened the amount of increase in his girth. I understand he was going to discuss this with Dr Horn.

Sally Morgan, the freelance journalist, who wrote two magazine articles about me and my micropenis, had this to say about my first book:

'I think it's very well written, David, and most amusing in places—full of anecdotes about yourself and other men with big/small ones. I particularly like the details about the details about Princess Margaret and her lover John Bindon, too'.

'But I would have edited out the details about how much you were paid by certain publications—and, if possible, have added some photos throughout the book to break it up a bit and illustrate the text. Hope this helps.'

I certainly value Sally's opinion and advice, and I was very pleased to read her compliments, but I also took on board her recommendations about things I can do to improve when writing a book of this nature.

On October 24, 2013, Sally phoned me to discuss certain things about this book. During our conversation, I asked her if she found it difficult to write about a taboo subject—penis size being among what must be the top three taboo subjects ever. I thought her first interview with me in 2002 would be the most difficult and embarrassing particularly as it was a face-to-face interview. The other interview, which took place in November 2005, I thought would be slightly easier because the interview was done over the telephone. Together with the fact that Sally knew most of my story by then anyway.

Sally confidently replied that she found writing the articles reasonably easy simply *because* the subject matter—penis size and penile enlargement surgery—was a taboo topic.

After our conversation, I still found it difficult to get my head around the fact how easy she found to write about my story. But then again, as Sally is such a talented writer and an excellent communicator, maybe I shouldn't have found it such a surprise that she could write so eloquently on the subject. I knew that she had done her research on this matter and that her articles were so professional to say the least. I'm hoping some of her ability will rub off on me!

If you look up the medical definition of a micropenis, it is described as an unusually small penis. This means an erect penis measuring smaller than about seven centimetres, or three inches. In infants a micropenis is classed as any penis that is less than three-quarters of an inch in length. This is considered significantly smaller than a normal male newborn's penis, which is between 1.1 and 1.6 inches in length when stretched gently.

As I've mentioned before one in two hundred men suffer from this condition. A man with a micropenis can have several problems, including difficulty urinating and having sexual intercourse. Fertility can also be affected. Some men with micropenises have a low sperm count, which results in infertility or decreased fertility.

Micropenis has a major impact psychologically as males with this condition have very low self-esteem and some even suffer from depression. This really rings true as far as I'm concerned. There may be some men who glory in the fact they have a tiny manhood—for example the guys that appeared on the Howard Stern radio show for the *Smallest Penis Contest*. What are these guys thinking?

What causes micropenis? According to some literature I've seen, it is caused by the male baby's failure to elongate after the first trimester of pregnancy. Elongation in the first trimester is described as follows: 'Minute ventilation is increased by 40 percent in the first trimester. The womb will grow to the size of a lemon by eight weeks.' The cause of this problem is thought to be a hormonal problem. Specifically, it is thought to be due to insufficient levels of testosterone, a male sex hormone.

The inadequate levels of testosterone may come as a result of inadequate production of testosterone during the second and third trimesters of pregnancy, or as a result of the unborn child lack of response to the testosterone produced.

Apparently, research carried out on Japanese patients and published in the *Journal of Clinical Endocrinology & Metabolism* found that mutations of the SRD5A2 gene can cause micropenis.

Researchers have also found that there may be a generic condition that makes boys more susceptible to the development of micropenis, and this condition is triggered by factors in the environment. Moreover, there is even further research to suggest that newborn-male external-genital malformations, such as micropenis, may be caused in part by environmental chemicals such as pesticides.

The condition is thought to affect one in two hundred males that are born. Telling these men, 'Size doesn't matter' is, to me, bordering on the offensive and, furthermore, is dishonest.

As you will have read in chapter four, there are now new surgical procedures to both lengthen and thicken the penis, which will function perfectly normally as a result. The micropenis can be increased in size to give the man suffering from the condition more confidence and self-esteem.

When such a man Googles the words, 'where can I get my penis surgically enlarged in London', (for example) the answers will be plentiful. This is where the man should be very selective and choose wisely.

For the purposes of this book, I made this very search query. One of the pages that came up was 'Penile Surgery London', their contact details being Tel: 0845 299 7774 and info@penilesurgerylondon. co.uk. The website claims, 'We specialise in penile surgery or penile enlargement. This procedure includes combining penile lengthening and penile thickening. Some people will address this surgery as manhood or love muscle enhancement', Lastly they state that they operate in London, Paris, and Brussels. All postoperative care and appointments are in London.

Micropenises

I will say that my book *Penoplasty: A True Story* is advertised by the clinic, and I'd be lying if I said I wasn't grateful to them. But as it says in the title, my story is true, so I do not feel any guilt in trying to promote my own book. As far as I'm concerned I suffered from micropenis and when I had the chance I tried to do something about. All I'm trying to do is tell those men out there who suffer from micropenis there is something you can do about it.

A man doesn't have to undergo the operation if he doesn't want to— but I think far too many people in the agony aunt profession, and some so-called medical experts, including doctors, are not truthful when it comes to male size and the penoplasty procedure. Perhaps some men who are underendowed will find that what they need is good counselling, and there's certainly no harm in that. However, that wouldn't have proved successful for me, and I suspect it wouldn't for the vast majority of men blighted by having a micropenis.

I've mentioned in chapter three the clinics where men can have the penoplasty/phalloplasty/penis enlargement procedure, and I came across another clinic in the United Kingdom. The following headline caught my eye, 'Penis Enlargement Surgery Nottingham/Penoplasty Clinic Nottingham'. Men were asked, 'Do you live in Nottingham, and are you considering Penis Enlargement surgery?' The article stated, 'We seem to be getting quite a few enquiries from Nottingham for penis enlargement surgery. Now, we are not reading too much into statistics, but it does appear that Nottingham men are not afraid to seek help if they believe that they have small penises. There has been a 45 percent rise in penis enlargement in the United Kingdom over the last couple of years.'

The following paragraph explains, 'Moorgate Aesthetics, based in the United Kingdom, are independent cosmetic surgery specialists in the field of penoplasty surgery. Because we are independent we are not tied to any particular hospital, clinic or surgeon.' Apparently this means that they can get you a very competitive price for your surgery, and at the same time they can give you choice in terms of your consultant and the hospital where you will have the surgery done.

Any interested man can phone the patient coordinator directly at 07714 795 869. Ask for David Mills, and he will be able to chat through any important questions you have about penis enlargement in the United Kingdom. The clinic informs men that a consultation will last around forty-five minutes to one hour and that you cannot consider penis enlargement without getting all the facts first. That seems very sensible to me. I obviously can't comment on the clinic or David Mills the surgeon, but the general set up and my gut instinct tell me it looks a promising place to consider having penoplasty done.

David Mills and Moorgate Aesthetics are based at 1 Sitwell Drive, Rotherham, South Yorkshire, S60 3AS and their telephone number is 0203 290 7789. Their website notes the following: 'London centre is the Mecca for penis enlargement surgery. It is one of those operations that are seldom discussed. There are not too many men willing to talk about it in public. However it's great to see some major national newspapers and magazines such as the *Sun*, the *Daily Mail*, the *Independent*, and a number of men's magazines such as *GQ* discussing the topic of penis enlargement surgery. Men want to know about this procedure and the more accurate the information that is available, the better for those looking to take the step.'

Now I want to get onto Lawrence Barraclough territory—I suppose I should apologise to the man in one respect because in my first book I misspelt his surname (Barrowclough instead of Barraclough). Sorry, mate, I didn't do it on purpose, but that's the only apology you're getting out of me. Now that I've got that out the way, I will repeat that I didn't think that much of the guy. Not because he's got a small penis, but the fact he edited my interview (on February 1, 2007) with him in such a way the cut that made it onto BBC3 screens was farcical. Any person watching would think I wasn't happy with my penis enlargement operations, when, in fact, I stated that my only regret was that I wished I had undergone my

Micropenises

first operation when I was twenty-two instead of at forty-two. He also gave a promise to Sally Morgan that he would allow her to interview him, and instead he 'blew her out' as the good people of East London would say. The man is a cad and a bounder as far as I'm concerned.

The territory Mr Barraclough occupied was, of course, a man with a very small penis considering having penile enlargement surgery. He then made not one but two documentaries (cockumentaries) about his life with a tiny penis. Some people thought he was very brave, some thought he was very mad, and I just thought he wanted to get from people whatever he could get for his TV programmes. My own opinion is that he had no intention of ever having penoplasty, he just wanted to make some television programmes and get his face and tiny penis on the nation's television screens.

Well, as mentioned in chapter seven, Mr Moote from across the pond also wanted to get his small penis recognised and mentioned in his own documentary, although it has to be said viewers never get to see his undersized penis, nor do they find out his exact size.

What's worse a man having a tiny dick or a woman having a pair of breasts that barely fill an AAA bra? Both Mr Moote and Mr Barraclough had their own agendas when informing the general public about their tiny todgers (to use a favourite word from the *Sun*). Mr Moote is an actor who presumably loves performing in front of the public, and Mr Barraclough is a television producer who loves getting his product out there for people to enjoy.

It's a pity that both British and American television viewers can't see a double act—the Moote and Barraclough show! Who has the biggest prick, or should it be the smallest? People could phone in to estimate to the nearest fraction of an inch who wins the booby prize!

I haven't seen Moote's cockumentary, but as you know I saw Barraclough's double-header on BBC3 and for a man with a small Hampton Wick (rhyming slang for prick if you're wondering) he really does talk a lot of balls.

MICROPENIS: The Long and Short of It

I've said this before and I'll say it again: most women, if they are honest, will say that penis size matters. More times than I can remember, I've heard on TV or read in newspapers or magazines that size does matter to women. Regrettably, I know from my own experience that being way too small creates a huge problem. That's not to say all of the women will tell a nice guy to his face that he is too small—but when push comes to shove, they will tell the truth and admit that size matters.

A certain Mr Jonah Falcon is famous for, reputedly, having the largest penis in the world, being nine and a half inches when flaccid and thirteen and half inches when erect. From a British point of view, he has appeared in a full spread article/photo in the *Sun* as well as on channel four's documentary/cockumentary *The Biggest Penis in The World*. Rumour has it that a large number of men with average-size penises feel inadequate compared to him. What, pray, should men with micropenises feel like? We know he's abnormal but so are the bottom 3 percent of men. That, possibly, makes tiny men feel twice as abnormal.

Now, I would like to inform you about Dr David Veale, who is a consultant psychiatrist in cognitive behaviour therapy at the South London Maudsley NHS Trust. He is also at the Priory Hospital in North London and sees patients privately as well.

I mention Dr Veale in relation to a report the *Sun* under the headline 'Big Guys' Willy Woe'. The story informed readers that British men worry about the size of their penises even if they are not small. It explained that experts believe one in three men suffer from 'small penis syndrome' where they have a sometimes debilitating fear of being rejected or laughed at.

The report explained that nearly two hundred men were measured at the Maudsley Hospital, in Camberwell, South London. In a flaccid state, they ranged from 2.8 inches to 7 inches and from 3.9 inches to 7.9 inches when erect.

On November 5, 2013, I wrote to Dr Veale about this article as well as about reports in greater detail on the Internet. I explained to Dr

Micropenises

Veale that as a man with micropenis I had no alternative but to go ahead with penoplasty when the procedure became available. I restated the fact that one in two hundred men suffer from the condition. I sent him my book *Penoplasty: A True Story*.

Dr Veale replied to me by e-mail. 'Very many thanks for sending me a copy of your book. I thought it was very interesting and very coura-geous to write about it. The research we are doing at present is on men who do not have a micropenis—some of them are in the lower range, and we are trying to understand some of their characteristics, compared to those who do not have concerns about their size.'

Dr Veale ended his reply by saying, 'We are recruiting a few more men for a trial we are doing on an extender, but I suspect it will be fin-ished by the time your new book is published. I am happy to send you the results of our studies when they are finally published. Good luck, David Veale.'

I replied, saying I would be very honoured if he could send me the details when his new trial has been completed.

Finally, I will say this. I have nothing but respect for Dr Veale because he took the time to read my book, but he also took time to let me know his views—and to inform me about his new trials concerning the pe-nile extender. The only other people to reply to my letter and enclosed book have been Deidre Sanders of the *Sun*, Dr Sheldon Burman, MD, Dr Harold Reed, Liz Gray of the London Centre for Aesthetic Surgery (LCAS), Sharon Mc Namara of the Belvedere Clinic, the producer of channel five's *Drastic Plastic* and, of course, Sally Morgan.

A large number of other people and organisations did not even bother to send me an acknowledgement. No more needs to be said oth-er than for me to use the phrase used by the notorious British punk rock band The Sex Pistols which is—'Never mind the bollocks, here's my sec-ond book.' Here's the truth and nothing but the truth so help me God.

For the record, I'm old enough to remember that the Sex Pistols won their day in court. People had complained about the title of their debut

MICROPENIS: The Long and Short of It

LP, *Never Mind the Bollocks Here's The Sex Pistols,* but when the case went to court, the lads from Shepherd's Bush and Finsbury Park had the right to call their record that because the word 'bollocks' can simply mean 'rubbish'.

CHAPTER TWELVE

The Penile Stretcher

It was only after I had watched myself in the documentary *Drastic Plastic* that I discovered there was a device called the Penis Stretcher that could carry on the good work that the surgeon had performed when he lengthened my penis. I would like to have seen my face as I watched this part of the programme!

The American surgeon who recommended the device to his patient, Anthony, was Dr Sheldon Burman. He informed Anthony that if he continued to use the stretcher over a long period of time, he would end up being huge. Bear in mind that Anthony was already eight inches when erect to begin with. Even if you are smaller than Anthony, it would be sweet music to a man's ears to be told that by the surgeon.

Dr Burman retired in April 2005, but he still performs a service for men who want larger penises by running the Penis Surgery Clinic on the Internet, where he offers advice. Regarding the penis stretcher he has this to say:

When human tissue is subjected to a stretching force it reacts by increasing its size. The tissue not only stretches, but its cells actually multiply, and new tissue is formed. The principle of traction is often used in modern medicine. For example, in order to cover burns, a tissue expanding device is placed under adjacent skin to stretch it.

MICROPENIS: The Long and Short of It

Orthopaedic surgeons exert traction upon bones to lengthen them. The Paduang tribe in Burma use rings to lengthen the necks of their 'Giraffe Women'. African tribesmen use wooden pieces to enlarge women's lips, and others hang weights to elongate ear lobes. Certain New Guinea tribesmen lengthen their male children's penises by attaching weights.

Based on these principles, a device for penile traction was designed. The device can be used with or without surgery. When used after it prevents shrinkage during the healing process. It also adds additional length. Without surgery, the stretcher will increase penis size, but it does so much more slowly than surgery. When properly worn, the stretcher is as comfortable as a wristwatch and cannot be seen under normal clothing. It is light and small—it weighs only a few ounces, and it can fit in your palm. It is flexible and collapsible. When worn properly, it fits easily into the inner surface of your thigh and cannot be seen underneath your tightest trousers—even blue jean cut-offs. The stretcher does not interfere with normal activities. You wear it 24/7 and only slip it off when you go to the bathroom, when you shower, when you have sex, and when you go through the metal detector at the airport. The amount of traction is adjustable by turning a couple of thumbscrews. When the tension is properly adjusted you will feel a gentle, not unpleasant pull on your penis.

The stretcher will work for any patient, regardless of age. The size increases are permanent. The average length gain in a recent series of sixty-two patients was between 0.143 and 0.248 inches per month in erection, and between 0.037 and 0.342 inches per month in a flaccid state in 95 percent of cases.

The length gain depends on how much tension you choose, how many hours a day, and how many weeks you wear it. There is no known limit to how much length you can gain. We have had patients who have worn it for seven years and have grown several inches.

The Penile Stretcher

The rate of length gain is essentially the same whether your penis is short or long to begin with. Stretching the penis is not like stretching a piece of taffy, which gets thinner as it gets longer. The increase in size involves the circumference as well as the length so that as the tension lengthens the girth widens proportionately. Using the stretcher does not interfere with erections, ejaculation, or sensation. The stretcher alone works more slowly than surgery, but it does work. Many patients will buy and wear their penis stretcher while they save money for their eventual surgery.

There was a report in *Science Daily* that hit the press thus:

Date: March 10, 2009

Summary: Men who used a penile extender every day for six months saw the length of their flaccid penis increase by 32 percent and their erectile function increase by up to 36 percent. Researchers at the University of Turin suggest the results were significant and patient satisfaction with the technique was high. The measurements were taken six months after the men had stopped using the device.

Men who wore a penile extender every day for six months were able to increase the flaccid length of their penis by up to 32 percent and their erectile function by up to 36 percent, according to an independent clinical study published in the March issue of BJU International.

Twenty-one highly motivated patients, with an average age of forty-seven, were enrolled and sixteen completed the twelve-month study, said consultant urologist Dr Palo Gontero. Having undergone psychosexual counselling, to make sure that the treatment would be beneficial, the men were asked to wear the AndroPenis device for between four and six hours a day for six months. The device comprises a plastic ring, two dynamic rods that produce the traction and a silicon band to hold the penis in place. The men were told to increase the traction from six-hundred grams in month one up to one thousand, two hundred grams in month six. Follow ups were performed in months one, three, six and twelve.

Some of the key findings included:

- The men's average flaccid penile length was 7.15 centimetres (2.82 inches) at baseline and had increased by 32 percent to 9.45 centimetres (3.72 inches) in month twelve.
- The men's average stretched penile length was 9.62 centimetres (3.79 inches) at baseline and had increased by 18 percent to 11.32 centimetres (4.45 inches) in month twelve.
- High satisfaction levels were reported in all categories except penile girth.
- Our study showed that the penile extender device produces an effective and durable lengthening of the penis, both in flaccid and stretched state.
- If these results are confirmed by further research, we propose that the device should be used as a front-line treatment option seeking a penile lengthening procedure.

Two years later on the *Health Day Daily News,* there was the headline, 'When Size Matters, Men Can Turn to Penile Extenders: Study'. The research was outlined as follows:

For men who believe size matters—and that their penises don't measure up—success can be found in certain nonsurgical penile lengthening treatments, a new study analysis by Italian researchers contends.

In a review of five evidence-based surgical studies of 121 men and six nonsurgical studies of 109 men published between 2000 and 2009, the researchers found that penile extenders—which stretch the organ over a period of months through traction—were the most effective among noninvasive methods.

The Penile Stretcher

Study coauthor Dr Paolo Gontero said urologists are constantly approached by men concerned about their penis size, despite the fact that many are average—with a flaccid length of four inches.

'However, most men complaining of inadequate penile size do have associated sexual problems even if their penile dimensions fall within the normal range', said Gontero, an associate professor of urology at the University of Turin.

Writing in an issue of the *British Journal of Urology International*, Gontero and his colleagues found that penile extenders work better than techniques such as vacuum devices, exercises, and Botox injections, and that psychological satisfaction is equally as important as any physical changes.

The men studied ranged in age from twenty-four to fifty-six and were followed between three and sixteen months. More than seventy of them used penile extenders, with six experiencing minor problems such as bruising, pain and itching. These devices yielded average flaccid length increases of between 0.2 inches and one inch, Gontero said, and men achieving better results noted their satisfaction.

'Application of progressive and constant traction forces is a very old-fashioned technique used by the ancestors and currently by some tribal populations to elongate the penis or the neck', he said.

Gontero noted that cognitive behavioural therapy might help build confidence in some men.

Long-term vacuum treatments did not appear effective, producing no significant physical changes after six months, Gontero said, but did provide a degree of psychological satisfaction.

My penile extender arrived in the post on March 24, 2005, the day before Good Friday, so it was a nice surprise and better than an Easter egg, if you ask me! I used it every day unless I was ill or was going away somewhere. Eventually the penile extender broke—or at least I think it broke; perhaps I used it too much. The first model had come with a small book of instructions, the front cover simply saying the JES extender (English).

Page two had line drawings of a small penis alongside another drawing of a larger penis. So far so good. Then on page three, there was the table of contents, with the first content being the Introduction. I was informed that the JES-Extender was designed and developed in Denmark by the medical specialist Jorn Ege Siana.

I read with great interest as the document informed me that the

JES Extender has been tested on patients who have obtained enlargement of the penis after the device is used in accordance with instructions. The enlargement is permanent and does not entail a narrowing of the circumference of the penis.

The test subjects achieved an average lengthening of the erect penis of 2.8 centimetres (24 percent) after a treatment period of three to four months. The treatment does not affect urination, sexual pleasure, or the ability to reproduce. Enlargement can only be obtained by daily usage of the device and the effect correlates with the number of hours of usage. The above-mentioned results were obtained after twelve hours' daily treatment over the period of three months.

The JES Extender can be used throughout the day for various periods of time. It is not necessary to wear the JES Extender for a long uninterrupted time to obtain results. As an example: two hours daily treatment for twelve months, will give the same final result as twelve hours daily for two months.

On the following pages, there came a description of the various components and instructions for assemblage of the JES Extender.

I did have to get a replacement for the JES Extender and so I contacted the London Centre for Aesthetic Surgery, 15 Harley Street, London

The Penile Stretcher

W1G 9QQ Tel: 020 7636 4272. I received my penile extender, which was now called Andropenis, within two days, as I recall. The leaflet that came with it showed a man in a black shirt with his arms crossed. Below him was a photograph of the Andropenis, along with an unfurled tape measure. The words written there, which looked very persuasive to me, said, 'Achieve a more satisfactory sex life'.

Inside the leaflet it explained the following: 'Medical applications', such as treatment for Peyronie's disease and nonsurgical treatment to increase penis length and girth. It continued with such claims as 'Scientifically proven', and recommended by prestigious urologists and andrologists worldwide. Andropenis, it said, is effective in 97.5 percent of cases. Only 2.5 percent did not obtain the desired result due to medical conditions.

The Andropenis has the following guarantees:

Andropenis is the only device of its kind on the market that has shown its complete and total safety.

Andromedical fulfils the international medical health requirements for clinical compatibility (e.g. it does not produce any skin irritation or hyper-sensitivity).

Andromedical holds a European standards approval mark (CE) as a type one medical product, which guarantees that there are no secondary side effects associated with the use of the use of this product.

On the next page the following experts endorse the device. Firstly, an American, Dr Wayne Hellstrom who is a Urology Professor and Director of Andrology at the University of New Orleans, United States of America. Professor Hellstrom states, 'The literature in a number of medical disciplines supports the concept of tissue expansion. The preliminary observations presented and published support the efficacy and safety of penile traction devices (such as Andropenis), for men with Peyronie's disease and in post operative penile surgical cases to maintain or gain penile length.'

MICROPENIS: The Long and Short of It

Secondly, French Urologist Dr Antoine Faix, who is also an Andrologist, Sexologist, and Director of the Mediterranean Centre for Sexology and Andrology says, 'I recommend this device to my patients (for both Peyronie's disease and penile lengthening). In my experience the results achieved are very encouraging.'

I adopted the approach that suited me. I wore the JES Extender for thirty minutes at a time for the first two weeks, before progressing to wearing it for an hour a day seven days a week. I gradually built this up an hour at a time until I wore it for seven or eight hours a day. I gradually saw an improvement over the next few months and by a year later, I would say, I had increased my penile length by an inch—which gave me greater confidence and self-esteem.

It does work! Of that there's no doubt. You have to stick at it and not expect to gain several inches over the first few weeks. It takes time and a man must be patient because if he isn't he will end up being disappointed—and we don't want that, do we, chaps? As that old saying goes, 'Steady as you go'. You will see the benefits if you adopt this method. Rome wasn't built in a day, and men who use this device must not rush things.

According to the figures on the Internet, the JES Extender has sold over one hundred thousand copies of the device, while the Andropenis has sold over three hundred and fifty thousand. These figures are very impressive, even more so when it's obvious that these figures will have to revised upwards over the coming years. I should also point out that Andropenis sells a device called Andropenis Mini, which is suitable for men with penises smaller than 3.2 inches (eight centimetres) when erect.

Lastly, I will mention some other devices that are available for men, women, and couples. If the bloke just doesn't want to have penoplasty or even try the penile stretcher, it's a free country, but if he does want to be bigger there are some other artificial ways to enlarge your manhood.

Freely available on the Internet are 'penis extensions' that the man can actually wear while making love to his wife or girlfriend. One item

The Penile Stretcher

is called the Tommy Gunn Be Him Cyberskin Penis Extension, which is actually moulded from Tommy Gunn's erect penis. As the advert says, 'you can turn your manhood into a perfect replica of his penis!' The measurement is quoted as eight and a half inches in length and is apparently priced at $16.40 plus $4.99 shipping. If you want this item simply find Delta Love on your home PC.

If, however, you want to be like Jeff Stryker, you can order his device from Amazon.com when you type in Health and Personal Care. Now please do not read this bit if you're easily offended or shocked—the advert blatantly says, 'Doc Johnson Realistic Jeff Stryker Cock with Balls'—ten and a half inches long and seven inches in girth.

If you want to stay with a British superstar, you can get a replica of Omar 'Big Willy' Williams' penis or, as the advert on the Delta Love says, 'A replica of his fully erect cock measuring ten inches in length.'

There are a few reviews on these websites from men who have worn these devices, mostly favourably, but there are some drawbacks, which are explained by the male customers. That said, most of the men—and women it must be said—do seem to like these toys, if that's what you call them. Although I have never tried these things out myself I see no harm in trying them out.

From a personal point of view, I'm still extremely happy that I opted for my five penis enlargement operations, and I'm very glad I used the Andro Penis device. Please note, no clinic or company has paid me to endorse these things.

CHAPTER THIRTEEN

'I'm Not Tempting Fate.'

Please go to the next chapter—the only impressive thirteen I've seen was Jonah Falcon's!

CHAPTER FOURTEEN

Odds and Ends

Here are some odds and ends about male penis size that's been in the news. It's rather amusing, or amazing, how the subject raises it's, shall we say, helmet from time to time.

On the same day (October 18, 2013) the article 'Big Guys' Willy Woe' appeared in the *Sun,* there was another article, entitled 'Condom for Super Manhood'. The story read, 'A *supercondom* said to give a firmer erection and to increase penis size has been approved for sale across Europe. Futura Medical said that Brussels bureaucrats are now satisfied the new offering is safe. The UK firm's product, known as CSD500, has been described as "Viagra in a condom". Futura claims it is "clinically proven to produce a firmer erection and increase penile size in healthy men". The condom also pledges to give women a "longer-lasting sexual experience". The award of the CE mark means CSD500 can be sold in several non-EU territories. City brokers CENKOS hailed the ruling as a countdown to a "condom revolution"'.

On the Internet I discovered that in December 2013, Futura signed a licensing agreement with Ansell Limited for the distribution rights to CSD500 in China. In December 2013, Futura also signed a licensing agreement with RFSU AB for the marketing and distribution of CSD500 in Sweden, Norway, Finland, and Denmark. CSD500 will also be available in a number of Middle Eastern and North African countries. Things certainly look big for CSD500.

Amazingly, although penis size wasn't directly mentioned, in the same edition of the *Sun,* the middle pages had an article entitled 'Five women who won't fib about their sexual history'. A larger headline underneath said, '*This* is the number of men we've slept with'. I will not print the surnames of the women who were interviewed and photographed—although they weren't shy in having their real names printed—the following numbers were given:

Charley has had two sexual partners.

Madison has had eighteen sexual partners.

Billie has had fifty sexual partners.

Becky has had 110 sexual partners.

Anna has had 180 sexual partners.

I'm not being judgemental about the five women interviewed; if other people want to be critical, it's up to them. However, I would put money on it that these women, with the possible exception of Charley, would definitely have preferences regarding penis size. Their experiences would certainly make it highly likely that they know what sizes they like and do not like.

Getting back to penis size and condoms, there was another article in the *Sun* on December 7, 2011, called 'Made to Pleasure', whose subheading was 'Condoms That Are Custom-Fit for Every Size'. Claiming to be an exclusive piece written by Emma Little (surely not!), we were informed that men could finally measure up in the bedroom—with the launch of tailor-made condoms. Ms Little informed us that 'figures showed almost half of users complained that standard brands are too small—or too big.'

As a result of this, a new firm, TheyFit, now offers ninety-five sizes, sold online at £6.99 for six. The boss, Joe Nelson, said: 'We have custom fit for clothes and shoes. Now we're applying it to something where great fit and comfort are even more critical to enjoyment.' The article

explained that customers could measure up at home with a chart printed from the website theyfit.co.uk, giving them a sizing code.

Meanwhile, on October 1, 2012, in the *Sun* we discovered that British
blokes have bigger willies than the French—but are dwarfed by men
from the Republic of Congo according to recent research. Apparently
our (British) national average is 5.5 inches, larger when compared to
Frenchmen's 5.3 inches, but according to the report men in the African
state are a 'massive 7.1 inches'. The least-endowed are Koreans, who average 3.8 inches.

The research was undertaken by Psychology Professor Richard
Lynn of Ulster University, who said that size is 'predictable' for most
nationalities.

Going back to August 2003, an article written by Gary Younge in
the *Guardian* was headlined, 'Size Does Matter, Jamaicans Decide'. The
story began, 'It was supposed to symbolise liberation and celestial rev-
erence in an independent Jamaica. Two naked seven-foot-high bronze
figures—a male and a female—looking skywards on a dome-shaped
fountain embossed with Bob Marley's lyrics 'None but ourselves can free
our minds.' But according to the statue's critics the artist is too light-
skinned, the male figure is too generously endowed, and both are, well,
too naked.'

It transpired that a columnist in Jamaica's *Daily Observer*, Lloyd Smith,
described the sculpture as 'a rape of our democracy'. However, another
writer ridiculed Renaissance sculptors for being not generous enough.
'Just because Europe's classical statues had small penises', argued Mark
Wignall, another *Observer* columnist, 'does not mean Jamaica must follow suit.'

The sculptor, Laura Facey Cooper, having attracted past criticism
for a near-naked and well-endowed carving of Christ, knew *Redemption
Song* would draw some flak but had no idea it would be so sustained.
Apparently many people did not have an issue with the figures' naked-
ness in general but the size of the man's penis in particular. The sculptor

used models and photographs and insisted, 'It is in proportion to the rest of the sculpture. I certainly didn't overplay it.'

Cooper remained unapologetic about the complaints that have come her way. She said, 'Both the male and female are very well-endowed in every possible way. It's an important part of life, and it's a wonderful part of life. I'm a wife, I have kids, and I enjoy that part of life.'

On a different aspect, although still about male size, I became aware that there had been a 'comedy drama', entitled *Hung*, about a school basketball coach who become rather short of money. As he had one advantage in life, a very large penis, he decided to make some money out of it by becoming a male escort—or put more bluntly, a prostitute. The programme ran from June 28, 2009 to December 4, 2011 on channel four, until the channel decided to pull the plug on it. I never saw the programme myself, but you can get the flavour of the series by reading the reviews on the Internet.

I really couldn't imagine a programme like this being made thirty years ago—certainly not forty years—because too many people would have complained. I know that there have been one or two serious documentaries made about real male prostitutes who 'service' female clients but that certainly wasn't thirty years ago. My first book covers this topic in some detail.

Regarding the acting profession, from time to time, the *Guardian* has interviewed Willem Dafoe—nothing wrong in that, of course. Once, however, Simon Hattenstone asked the actor if the rumours were true that he had Hollywood's biggest penis. When Stuart Jeffries interviewed Dafoe in June 2013, he returned to the subject again and asked him, 'Do you?' Apparently Dafoe laughed obligingly before heading off to rehearsal. He replied, 'I don't really work in Hollywood any more.' Jeffries last words were, 'Which, you'll notice, isn't a denial.'

I think most people of a certain age are aware of an item of male clothing called the 'willy warmer'.

Odds and Ends

A Croatian seamstress, Radmila Kus, has revealed she is struggling to cope with the huge demand for the latest product—her very own range of willy warmers. Rudmila said she just can't keep up with demand after launching her bespoke men's product, and has had to recruit a small army of knitters in a bid to increase production.

This traditional piece of European clothing was historically used by Croats on exceptionally long horse rides or while working as shepherds. They were especially popular in Croatia's remote Mrkopalj mountain region, where wives knitted the protection to help their husbands cope with the area's freezing weather. Radmila makes the made-to-measure garments with the help of additional staff. She revealed, 'If people are shy, they can provide me with their measurements.' These garments are also worn in Norway and Denmark.

In the late twentieth and early twenty-first centuries, willy warmers have usually been made as novelties and joke gifts rather than to serve a functional purpose. In 1939, while filming *Gone with the Wind*, Clark Gable received a present of a hand-knitted genitalia warmer from Carole Lombard. In the 1950s, Joan Crawford knitted a 'cock sock' as a parting present for Porfirio Rubirosa.

I remembered Porfirio Rubirosa's name from a magazine article I read some years ago. I've seen on the Internet an article from *Vanity Fair* about 'The Legend of Rubirosa'. The article noted, 'In the fifties, jet-set Porfirio Rubirosa was the ultimate man's man, with his polo, Ferraris, and macho adventures. But what made the Latin diplomat truly unforgettable were his women—an endless parade including Barbara Hutton, Doris Duke, Ava Gardner, and Jane Mansfield—and the physical endowment that enslaved them.

'The late Truman Capote described Rubi's (Rubirosa's nickname) principal endowment in his unfinished novel, *Answered Prayers*, as an "eleven-inch cafe-au-lait sinker as thick as a man's wrist". When asked to compare Rubi's member to a writer's size-eleven shoe, one of his paramours glanced at the shoe, merely shrugged, and said, "Rubi's was bigger."'

In one article it was written that, 'His real legacy to the world was that, in certain restaurants when people want a pepper mill, they still require a Rubirosa.' This is because his penis was said to be as big as a pepper mill.

I've mentioned before the documentary shown on channel five *A Girl's Guide to 21st Century Sex*, where a couple are actually filmed having sexual intercourse with a camera inside the woman's vagina and a camera attached to the man's penis. The man's name, believe it or not, is Stefan Hard! You couldn't make it up.

On the Internet one can find all manner of stuff concerning the male appendage. If you are interested or shall we say curious you can see the following websites: Your Guide to Men's Health Issues, which shows penis pictures where you can rate the guy's penis size (a guy over eight inches received 92 percent of the votes—well there's a surprise!), Soft Hard Gallery Erection Photos; Penis Pictures Galore, Photos from Measure Up and Snap your Chap, which was originally shown on Embarrassing Bodies on channel four here in the United Kingdom.

As you may be aware, the 'Snap Your Chap' came from none other than Lawrence Barraclough who is the smart-arse TV producer who tried to persuade all the men in the world—straight and gay—that penis size just doesn't matter at all. It goes without saying that all the billions of women in the world never give penis size a second thought—believe that if you must!. Dear Lawrence seems to live on a different planet to me. I'm pretty sure the whole concept of 'Snap Your Chap' was to reassure all the men in the world that even if your penis didn't measure even a fraction of an inch you could be considered 'normal'. I've looked at the photos on 'Snap Your Chap' and sorry to say 99.9 percent of the dicks would still make me feel inadequate if my size was that of my micropenis years.

Odds and Ends

Lastly, I'll go back to the problem pages in our daily popular newspapers—or red tops as they are called in Britain. One letter was from an eighteen-year-old man to 'Dear Deidre' in the *Sun* explaining that his willy was not any bigger than when he was three. Furthermore, he said he wasn't a bad-looking guy but that all his friends laughed at the fact that he's only two inches long when erect. He was worried that a doctor would also laugh if he went to see him. Also, a couple of girls had laughed in the past, so he kept away from women now.

The reply stated that Deidre felt his story was very sad, but that he should really go to see his doctor. Then came the regimented, to me at least, 'advice' where Deidre said, 'Whatever your inches, there are loads of sensitive, loving women out there who are not obsessed with size.' In my book the young man should be referred to a consultant urologist at the very least—preferably one experienced in enlargement techniques. The young man is unfortunately in the club that no man wants to be in, namely the guy who happens to be the one man in two hundred who has an abnormally small penis. That's a fact and no amount of soft soap and kind words are likely to make the young man feel any better.

On the other hand (or penis), a twenty-three-year-old man wrote to Deirdre, informing her that the size of his penis was getting him down. Yet another man worried about his small (tiny) size? Not a bit of it; this was a guy telling us that when people meet him they don't look at his face but at the bulge of his jeans. My first thought was, I should be so lucky! We then learn that his penis is nearly thirteen inches long. Are we meant to feel sorry for him? He admits to a 'silly amount of partners' because of his size. Up until I was thirty, I had a 'silly amount of partners', and if you read my first book, you would know my figure was zero. Yes, zero, and I was not exactly jumping up and down with joy, I can tell you.

Then we discover that he gets older women 'coming on' to him, which makes him feel cheap. When I was twenty-three, if older women had come on to me, I would have felt like a million dollars. Some people don't know how lucky they are. Deirdre replies that lots of men would would envy him. No, Deirdre, I don't *think* I would envy him; I *know* I would. She ends by telling him to try on different styles of jeans and trousers in a department store, so he can work out what suits him best. Then the knockout blow is that he should wear a different pair of strides (trousers!) that leaves him less vulnerable to 'gawpers'. Saints preserve us that this is the same newspaper that for the last decade or so has printed countless stories about women preferring well-hung men. Within these very pages there are reports about researchers who have established that women like to gawp at men's bulges. If women don't do it consciously they certainly do subconsciously.

CHAPTER FIFTEEN

There Are Other Things to Worry About

There's absolutely no doubt that from the time I was thirteen years old until August 13, 1996, when I had my first penis enlargement operation, I was worried sick about my 'one-inch stump'. No amount of 'soft soap' from well-meaning agony aunts, friendly agony uncles, or all those do-gooders who trot out the usual old clichés such as, 'It's not the size, it's what you do with it' will make a man with a 'one-inch stump' feel any better about himself. When a guy, belonging to that one-in-two-hundred club, who possesses a micropenis, hears that rubbish no wonder he feels annoyed.

I felt like screaming at the last problem page or documentary I had just seen trotting out the mantra, 'Don't worry about your small penis.' What kind of butterball do you take me for? When a boy has read a book about puberty, which tells him that his penis will grow longer and thicker as he grows up so that eventually his genitals will then distinguish him from a young boy, he is full of hope. But what happens when his penis does not grow at all, and he clearly sees that other lads are growing towards adulthood, and he isn't?

The only thing that an undersized boy will grow, regrettably, will be a huge inferiority complex, which will be made worse because the other lads will give him a horrible nickname such as I was given—'Little Dick' and 'Half Inch'. Thanks for nothing Mother Nature. How sick I used to feel when I heard about women who liked men who could 'completely fill them up'. Or, as I heard a woman say, 'Long and thick does the trick.'

When men have phoned me up via the Belvedere Clinic or the Mayfair Clinic, and some of them have confided in me that they too have been affected by the micropenis condition, I can tell the pain they've suffered. Not all of these men have been that small, some being slightly below average but not tiny and other guys being Mr Average—six inches or thereabouts. But all had legitimate reasons for wanting to be bigger.

As I mentioned in chapter twelve, the documentary *Drastic Plastic* informed viewers about Anthony, who was already eight inches while erect but still wanted to be bigger. We have to accept that some men, although already well endowed, want to possess an even bigger package.

At this point I have to tell you all that, as I've got older—certainly since having my first penoplasty operation when I was forty-two—there are indeed other things to worry about. Without doubt, health worries have played a part in my life. More and more high levels of medication have given me more side effects than I know what to do with. If you're squeamish, don't read the next few paragraphs. Here are some of my medical problems and side effects I've had for the last ten years:

A). Diarrhoea and constipation—unfortunately, you can suffer from both in one week. This is brought about by my intake of several drugs—some episodes are 'overflow diarrhoea'.

B). Stomach ulcers caused by taking Naproxen for ten years (1991 to 2001), which I took for migraines and background headaches. From 2013 I've been taking them again for arthritis.

C). Arthritis in both my knees and right hip—regrettably, this has been caused by age.

D). Memory lapses combined with physical clumsiness, brought on by my large cocktail of drugs.

There Are Other Things to Worry About

E). Suffering from depression—not only because I had a micropenis, but because my mother passed away in 1999 from cancer, looking like a concentration-camp victim. My antidepressants (also taken for my migraines and acting as sedatives) leave me with a dry mouth that's actually painful, with my tongue sticking to the roof of my mouth. I have been diagnosed as suffering from an adjustment disorder, prolonged depressive reaction.

F). A chronic infection of the prostate which frightens the life out of me.

There are other health problems, but the above will do for now. The last one mentioned is a medical condition called chronic prostatitis, which was only diagnosed because of the knowledge of a senior consultant urologist I saw at a seminar in my then GP's surgery in February 2013. Even after having several tests before this, with two separate consultant urologists, no correct diagnosis was made.

I was first aware of my condition in May 2010 when I was masturbated by my wife and found to my horror that my semen—which was tiny in quantity—was the colour of strawberry jam. My heart was in my throatwhen this occurred because it had never happened to me before. It shows how naive I was because I had never heard of this problem.

I made an appointment to see a doctor—not my own GP, because I had been seeing him for so many other health problems—I wanted to see someone else. Not only that, but for some unknown reason, I knew I would be embarrassed to see my own GP. I was aware of a general message in the media for the last decade or so that was, 'don't die of ignorance', so at least I made an appointment to see a doctor, even though it was one I had never seen before.

The male doctor I saw was very understanding and could see how scared I was. He decided it was advisable that I had blood, urine, and semen tests to see what the problem was. In fact, I had numerous tests, and though I had traces of blood in my urine (not seen by the human eye), and in my semen (very often called spunk), I was told that my tests were clear.

Later on, I had some very sensitive tests. One of the tests was to investigate my bladder to see why I was passing blood in my urine. It was one of the most embarrassing things I've ever had to go through in my life, however necessary it was. The procedure was called a cystoscopy, and I was ushered in to a room by a female nurse. Shortly afterwards, another female nurse entered and then requested I take off my trousers and pants. I then got on an examination table and did what you're supposed to do in circumstances like that—I laid back and thought of England, not forgetting Scotland, Northern Ireland, and Wales!

The urologist came in and then explained he was going to examine my bladder by using a flexible cystoscope to see if I had any problems. I had the two nurses standing either side of me as the male urologist started to insert the cystoscope into my penis—he did this after using some substance (a gel?) to ease the device in to the opening of my penis. It didn't feel horrendous as I thought it would be, but then again, it certainly wasn't pleasant.

All the time I was aware that the two nurses were standing over me and watching the procedure being done by the urologist. All I could do was shut my eyes as tightly as I could. Boy, did I wish I were somewhere else, enjoying a nice meal and a cup of tea.

My experience in front of the cameras for the channel five programme *Drastic Plastic* helped me in some way get through this ordeal, with this instrument travelling through my penis. I obviously didn't have over one million viewers watching me like I did on television, but please believe me when I say that without that experience, helped by a fantastic TV producer, I don't think I would have gone through with the cystoscopy. I think I would have made the decision not to go to the hospital. Instead, I would have worried myself sick about why I was having blood in my urine and semen. I'm a terrible coward at the best of times, and

There Are Other Things to Worry About

I would have just thought to myself that whatever the problem was, if it killed me, so what.

I continue to have blood in my semen—and I still worry about that to this day. Not only that, but when I had to take a sample of my semen (which still the colour of strawberry jam) into my GP's surgery, I had to hand it over to one of the female receptionists. As I gave it to her, in hushed tones she remarked, 'There isn't much for them to do the test.' It's one of those times when you want the ground to open up and swallow you whole.

This is one of the things that I've always worried about: I've never produced a lot of semen, even when I was a young man, and alongside my tiny size, this caused me so much anguish. I'm sure Mr Average (six inches long and five inches in girth) produces much more semen than I've ever managed.

What's more, when I come my semen only dribbles out—I've never really spurted out my semen like I would love to. Again Mr Average would, I'm sure, put me to shame, never mind British porn stars like Omar 'Big Willy' Williams or Danny Dong, who apparently is not only huge in size but can ejaculate a huge amount a very long way. Thanks so much, I thought; that really makes me feel good about myself!

A few days after the cystoscopy, I felt very ill, and one night at about 1:00 a.m. I had to go to the toilet, and to my dismay, I was peeing blood—the colour of claret, I would say. My urine was this horrible claret colour for the next three days—my wife had to take time off from work to look after me. My GP prescribed antibiotics to clear up the infection. When I saw her a week or two afterwards, she explained that the actual procedure where the urologist examined my bladder gave me the infection. Even with the best of hygiene in the hospital and in the room where they did the procedure, it still leaves the patient open to infection. She explained that no object normally passes up my penis and into my bladder.

MICROPENIS: The Long and Short of It

I've had other health worries, such as a nasty large toenail on my left foot, which has given me problems since the early 1990s. After wearing a brand-new pair of Dr Martens boots to a concert, both my large toenails ended up being totally black. I had worn the boots all day and continued to wear them at the concert, and by the time I got home it was about 1: 00 a.m. My GP at the time decided to take off my large right toenail completely and take a section of my large left toenail away. It was as unpleasant as it sounds.

My large left toenail has caused me problems ever since. In 2010, after inspecting my toenail over a period of time, my GP decided to refer me to a local hospital to investigate. I was so naive that I didn't realise how potentially dangerous this problem could be. It was only after reading the letter and enclosures from the hospital that I realised that my GP was worried it may turn cancerous. It put the fear of God into me. Luckily, my appointment with the dermatologist came round soon, and he was a plain speaking consultant to say the least. After a quick inspection of my toenail, he said there were two things he had to tell me. Firstly, the toenail was 'knackered', but secondly, it wasn't cancerous. I was so relieved I wanted to shout for joy. You have to go through that kind of worry to understand how much a few reassuring words can be.

What I'm trying to say at the end of my book is that there are many other things to worry about other than the size of your penis. As I've gotten older, and my health has caused me so many concerns, that fact has become apparent. However, I'd be the biggest liar on this planet if I said penis size wasn't important, because it damn well is. A friend of mine has recently said to me that I'm 'getting on a bit'. That might be so, but I still don't want to die a horrible death.

Although age and the passing time tells me that there are indeed other things to worry about, recent events remind me of my micropenis anxiety. A poll undertaken by YouGov in Britain asked the all-important question, Does penis size matter? Apparently 52 percent of the UK adult population did not think that 'when it comes to sex, a man's penis size matters', while 38 percent think it does. Amongst women, 57 percent disagreed with the statement, but a large proportion (35 percent) said that size does matter. Men were evenly divided, with 42 percent who said size mattered, while 48 percent said it doesn't.

Did these figures offer me any comfort?—not on your life. These figures, in fact, prove agony aunts and sexperts are miles off course with their boring old clichés that size doesn't matter. Their point of view would be true if it was the case that 99.9 percent of men *and* women said size didn't matter. But these figures prove strongly that large numbers of men *and* women say it does. Once again, I will state the bleeding obvious (a bit of Basil Fawlty) that if the men were unfortunate enough to suffer from having micropenises, and women were unfortunate enough to have boyfriends with that problem, I think the figures would be about 90 percent or more saying that size definitely matters. After all, they would just be telling the truth.

There has been a case recently concerning the publicist, Max Clifford, who is facing various charges of sexual offences against underage girls, where in the question of his penis size was raised (sorry, no pun intended). According to the evidence some claimed his penis was 'freakishly small', while some claimed it was 'enormous'. In court it was recorded that Clifford's own doctor measured his penis, and it was discovered Clifford's penis, when flaccid was five-and-a-quarter inches long. We all know things are relative, but I can honestly say that compared to my one-inch stump (only half an inch when cold) Mr Clifford dwarfs me. The court heard Clifford's penis is 'average'. Perhaps you can understand why I worried so much about my tiny appendage.

My first book was dedicated to the one in two hundred men who suffer from micropenis, and to be honest, I want to dedicate this second book to them as well. It's one of the clubs a man wouldn't want to belong to. There's only one thing I would go back to my one-inch stump for. What is that, you wonder? This to me is a no-brainer, because if I could have my mother back with me, free from cancer, even I would put up with the horrors of a micropenis. To see her face knowing that she's got a beautiful granddaughter would be Heaven indeed. Mind you, I only fathered a child after I had my penis enlarged, which certainly enhanced not only my size and confidence but also my performance. Quite a few people would deny that but I say different. This book is therefore still dedicated to the one-in-two-hundred club. Although as I've mentioned above, there are dozens of other problems that can put the fear of God into you. But regarding penis size, this book's for the needy, *not* the greedy!

'A Little Bit of What You Fancy Does You Good'

It struck me after I had thought I had finished this book that there were a few extra things I wanted to include, so here's chapter sixteen.

There's an old song—well, to be truthful, a very old song—that states that a little bit of what you fancy does you good. Research has found that men who have sexual intercourse three or more times a week will halve their risk of having a stroke or a heart attack.

Furthermore, medical and scientific research shows that regular lovemaking slows down the ageing process and keeps you looking young. In addition, it improves your immune system and reduces stress. What could be more natural and, for most men, pleasurable?

The problem I have with this is my concern for the one in two hundred men who suffer from micropenis. They would benefit from regular lovemaking just like Mr Average, but the vast majority of men with micropenises will have performance anxiety. They would also be anxious about lack of pleasure for their partners, which would regrettably outweigh any of the wonderful bonuses mentioned above.

I recently read a forum online for the women's magazine *Cosmopolitan*, where the following statement appeared, 'My friends and I were talking and have decided that guys with smaller penises [come] quicker than those with bigger ones. Apparently it is to do with more nerve endings in a smaller area.' This all seems to make complete sense to me, and it's something I read about years ago—and I do mean years ago, probably about twenty years ago. It was research done by doctors and their staffs. How did that make me feel? I felt bloody awful, to be brutally honest, although it does all stack up. Before my operation my few opportunities of lovemaking with my first sexual partner resulted in my coming within five seconds. It's not something that made me feel good about myself.

It was lucky for me that after my first operation, at which time I was married to my second and only other partner, my stamina in bed improved, which made me feel better. That said, I would still love to last much longer than I do, but I am grateful for small mercies. I know there are supposed to be certain techniques that you and your partner can employ so the man can 'learn' to last longer. Perhaps the techniques really do help some men with this problem, but I've read that the majority of these unfortunate men are still left wanting.

What really makes my blood boil are the condescending experts (are they really experts?) who say to men with small penises they should make do with what nature (or God?) has given them. These so-called 'experts' would no doubt trot out this garbage to the men who suffer from micropenis. I really can't stomach this bog-standard type reply, which, to me, shows these 'experts' to be both lazy and dishonest.

A heart-warming story appeared in the *Daily Mirror* newspaper on April 23, 2014, which concerned a man who suffered a botched circumcision when he was a child. The man, Mike Moore, became the first person in the world to conceive a baby with a totally reconstructed penis.

He was just seven years old when doctors had to amputate most of the organ, which became infected after a routine surgery went wrong. It led to years of bullying, eventually the breakdown of his first marriage, and a long struggle with depression. But he became the proud parent of a son named Memphis with his new wife, Heather.

'A Little Bit of What You Fancy Does You Good'

In 2007, he flew over two thousand miles to California to visit a surgeon, Dr Gordon Lee. Although Mr Moore had already had three attempts to rebuild his penis, these proved to be unsuccessful. However, Dr Lee took skin from Mr Moore's thigh to make the organ, and this time it worked. The surgeon said, 'His story is, as far as I know, a first in the world for a totally reconstructed penis to go and have a baby.'

The couple wanted to have the baby naturally, but after months of trying, they turned to artificial insemination using his sperm—and his second wife got pregnant. Apparently they are now trying for another child.

From a different standpoint, there was a terrible story in the British press about a man in Middlesborough, who had his penis chopped off in what appeared to be a dispute over a woman. The distressed man was put into an induced coma after being found searching the undergrowth, to the side of the A66, looking for his shorn manhood.

The Internet gave a comprehensive list of the questions most asked about men who have had their manhood chopped off. The first question was, 'How much does it hurt?' It's never happened to me, but I suspect it's incredibly painful. The official answer was, 'Acute—almost certainly blinding pain.' It was stated that severing the penis without removing the testicles is said to cause intense frustration, since all urges and sex drive come from the testicles, and, short of the penis, the unfortunate man in question has no way to satisfy them.

The next question was, 'Can it be reattached?' The answer given was, 'If the shorn penis can be reattached via surgery, there is apparently no reason why people cannot go on and live a fruitful and relatively normal life.' A Chinese study of fifty men who underwent reattachment surgery found that all but one achieved full functionality again. Remarkably, that was the case even if the operation required reattaching both tissue and bone.

MICROPENIS: The Long and Short of It

The next question was 'What if reattachment isn't possible?' The reply was, 'In some cases reattachment is not an option and a new penis, made from tissue grafted from another part of the body, must be made.'

'Can you still have sex?' was the next question, which is obviously a very important issue; in the Chinese study all but one of the patients recovered full functionality with some reportedly going on to father children after the removal. With the reattachment option a manufactured penile implant is needed for an erection to take place, but ejaculation is either not possible or not with as much force.

What's this got to do with a poor sod with a tiny micropenis? I, for one, would say that these terribly underendowed men would actually feel like their poor excuses for penises had suffered under a knife. At least a man who has had part or all of his penis cut off has an excuse for lacking in the manhood department. What's a man to say when Mother Nature (or God) has sold him tragically short? Please don't think I'm in any way underestimating the horrendous act of a man having his penis chopped off. But a man who has very little penis to speak of, due to Mother Nature's cruelty, should also have some compassion and sympathy in my humble opinion.

Another subject I want to return to is the ever growing list of TV programmes that leave very little, if anything, to the imagination. My previous book covered this topic in some detail, but I think it is worthwhile pursuing this discussion. I am aware of the programme *Embarrassing Bodies*, which has been aired on channel four and does not pull any punches. I would love to know the answer to this question—are we growing more accustomed to explicit cameras shots of genitalia? Or have we, the viewing public, just reached a point where we have seen so much of it that it has desensitised our thoughts and emotions? It's corny I know, but is it a case of, 'If you've seen one you've seen them all'? Has the saturation point been reached?

Looking at *Embarrassing Bodies* on the Internet, there's a series of penises—numbering in their dozens—and lo and behold we find out

'A Little Bit of What You Fancy Does You Good'

that it's none other than Lawrence Barraclough who provided the photographs with his Snap Your Chap gallery. Couldn't channel four produce a selection of dicks to call their own? Why did they have to go to Mr Lawrence 'I've got a small one, but I know how to use it' Barraclough?

At least *Embarrassing Bodies* was honest enough to explain the genuine problems caused by buried penis and micropenis. The problem was explained as follows, 'Believe it or not, it's thought that up to one out of every two hundred men is born with what's medically known as a micropenis. It's an exclusive club and members (pun intended) need to be less than seven centimetres (two and three quarters inches) to join. Most of these men have trouble urinating and having sexual intercourse.' Three cheers for a television programme about sex—particularly about penis size—that speaks honestly about a taboo subject.

Channel four even explained that penoplasty (phalloplasty) can and does help these men—whatever next!

Another channel four programme that pretended to talk sense about sensitive issues (whisper it, these issues concerned penis size) but ended up trotting out the same tired old clichés that every penis is normal—this programme was *Sex Education*. This really made me want to throw up. Anna 'I'm an expert on all sexual matters' Richardson and her colleague gave the impression, without actually saying it, that a bloke with a one-inch penis and another with a foot-long penis would be both considered 'normal'. Both Ms Richardson and her sidekick had the brass neck to say to these fourteen- and fifteen-year-old schoolchildren that all penises regardless of size are all 'normal'. What would you do with people like this?

Ms Richardson loved the shock tactics of showing her 'Erection Gallery' where men—all of whom were photographed below the waist—had their flaccid penises shown alongside their erect penises. She worked herself into a lather by pointing out the smaller penises were 'growers', and the larger penises didn't grow so much. She pointed out that the first guy—who had a three-inch flaccid penis—doubled in size to become a six-inch erection. What dear Anna didn't mention was that the guy had an extremely thick girth—thick when flaccid and even thicker when erect.

A guy with a short penis, she pointed out in glee, trebled his size when erect, whereas a guy with a very long penis 'only put on one and a half inches when erect'. The problem for me—do I have to spell it out again?—is that all these men would have put me to shame before I had my penoplasty procedures. If the aim of her Erection Gallery was to make all the school lads feel more confident—as well as a few million adult males—she might well have failed miserably with a large number of the guys watching this programme. In fact, I read a number of comments from some lads after the video, and it was evident that a number of them did not agree with Ms Richardson. It's good to know that the lads publicised their disagreements with the so-called experts.

Of course, a number of men and school children may well have agreed with Anna and the gang. It's a free country, and your phallus is your own business, but what I will say is that I heard a very attractive woman comment that the cliché, 'Size doesn't matter, it's what you do with it', has been trotted out so much many women have been brainwashed to actually believe it. Needless to say, the very attractive woman in question believes that's a load of nonsense. She knows size does matter, although I don't think she wants every guy below five inches to be sentenced to twenty years hard labour. She would, however, agree with Julie Burchill that not all blokes are born equal. That's a statement of fact, or as Basil Fawlty of *Fawlty Towers* would say, 'Why don't we put you on *Mastermind*—subject the bleeding obvious.'

Before I leave the issue of adult subject matters on television, there was a sensible debate about this on the BBC programme *Breakfast* in May 2014. It was stated that there has been an official TV watershed since the 1950s. Earlier in this book I have obviously discussed the watershed in some detail, with comments from the producer of *Drastic Plastic* explaining her point of view. The watershed, from my point of view, has been

'A Little Bit of What You Fancy Does You Good'

gradually eroded over the last few decades. One person pointed out that children (or anyone else for that matter) can see programmes of an adult nature on 'catch-up' television. Other ways for underage children to see these programmes are the following: using computers (at home or in someone else's home), laptops, mobile phones, and any number of other technical devices that I have very little knowledge of. Nowadays most young children can obtain any manner of programmes/images from their modern devices.

Apparently children, using these sophisticated devices, can not only view postwatershed TV programmes but also see hard-core pornography. How governments, parents, guardians, or any other custodians of morality can stop children viewing these things I really don't know. Have any readers of this book got any ideas?

Women like a bit of what they fancy just as much as men. They like good-looking men, but men who aren't too vain and self-obsessed. Generally women like blokes who are clean, honest, trustworthy, and caring. This might sound a little bit yucky, but I really do believe women appreciate these things. If a man has some money in the bank, that's not going to present a problem either!

If we are going to be hardnosed about other things, many women like men who are not sexist, not homophobic, and not racist, but one thing women do definitely appreciate (as recent research has shown) is a well-hung man. If that sounds sizeist (if there's such a word), too bad! You're not going to tell me millions of men do not appreciate curvaceous women—we are all born with a pair of eyes (not counting the poor people who are unfortunately blind) so we are visual beings. Face up to the fact that many straight women like the look of a large penis; this might be at a subconscious level, but it's still true. A little bit of what you fancy does you good.

According to Carole Cadwalladr in the *Observer* of May 4, 2014, women do not like men such as Max Clifford, who was mentioned earlier in this book, and who was sentenced to eight years in prison. Ms Cadwalladr wrote in her piece that Clifford was 'undone by his need to dominate, to boast of his affairs.' Carole Cadwalladr interviewed Clifford in 2005 and discovered what a thoroughly manipulative and unpleasant person he was.

At Clifford's trial, the issue concerning the size of his penis became a matter for the jury. Ms Cadwalladr said, 'I went back to a story I wrote in 2006 to check what he'd told me on the subject. Clifford is "impervious to criticism", I wrote. He doesn't even attempt to justify himself "because I can't." The only thing he'd really mind, he tells me is if someone said he was rubbish in bed. Or "that I had a small willy."'

She continued, 'It's a measure of the desperateness of his situation that to Clifford, his penis, his "willy" as he'd have it, which his doctor claimed was "within the average range for a Caucasium male of Mr Clifford's age", had to be one of the main lines of his defence.'

This is me speaking now—in the court it was confirmed that Mr Clifford's flaccid penis measured five and half inches. This is average? I'm here to say how inadequate I felt reading this information, and what a big-headed bastard Mr Clifford sounds to me.

Mr Clifford informed her during their interview that 'Nearly everybody I've ever known has affairs. Nearly every journalist I've ever met has affairs. I haven't met one, in forty-odd years, who hasn't. It's not that I think they are; I know they are!' It was a delight that Ms Cadwalladr replied in her Observer piece, 'Well, no, Max, you don't, actually.'

Ms Cadwalladr continued, 'I remember one year, during these times, when the *News of the World* won newspaper of the year at the Press Awards. I was at the awards at the *Observer* table, sitting next to an American journalist, Sarah Lyall, who was writing for the online magazine, *Slate*. The evening, she wrote was "like a soccer match attended by a club of misanthropic inebriates"; the tone set by Sir Bob Geldof, there to present a prize to the *Sun*, "I've just been down at the bog" he said. "And it's true that rock stars do have bigger knobs than journalists."'

'A Little Bit of What You Fancy Does You Good'

Back to Ms Cadwalladr, 'Knobs, willies, cocks. There's been a turbocharged masculinity at the heart of British newspaper culture for decades. And, so it turns out, to abuse the trust not just of the British public, but of vulnerable underage girls too. This competition that is British public life, the need to prove the size of your cock, the expectation that public figures are corruptible, that all people, everywhere, are simply out for themselves, this idea that life is, at its core, a willy-waving contest, this has not gone. This is still here. This is Max Clifford's world and we live in it still.'

Strong words from Carole Cadwalladr but although Clifford is still with us, at least he was given a prison sentence. I agree that 'willy-waving' contests do go on in all of our culture, businesses, private, and public enterprises, and the worst offender is often rock culture. How we stop it I simply don't know.

If I were ever lucky enough to have a large penis, I honestly—hand on my heart—would not go around seeking affairs with women. I would, hopefully, have enough decency and common sense to have a one-on-one relationship with a woman who was my equal or indeed my superior. I couldn't think of anything more satisfying than that. That said, if I was a single bloke not in a relationship, and I was offered 'employment' as a male stripper, for example—given that I was well hung, good-looking, and had the confidence to stand fully naked in front of a room full of screaming women—I would take up the offer. I would also take up the position of someone like Joel from Melbourne (see my first book) if the opportunity arose.

The *Sunday Mirror's* TV critic, Kevin O'Sullivan, had a real go at channel four's *Embarrassing Bodies* live from the clinic on April 20, 2014. Under the heading 'No more willy-nilly doctors', he said, 'The nation's favourite purveyors of unconscionable voyeurism...' Mr O'Sullivan continued, 'If tawdry TV medics Christian Jessen, Dawn Harper and Pixie McKenna choose to earn a living persuading poor saps to show us their bent willies on telly, good luck to them. But don't pretend that making laughingstocks of people with filmically disgusting diseases is some sort of essential service. As always, after their hapless patients' unfortunate ailments had graced the screen (live!), caring Chris and the gang simply referred them to specialists. Random question: is there such a thing as the hypocritical oath?'

Do I think I was treated like a sap when I appeared on channel five's *Drastic Plastic*? The honest answer is no—but perhaps some of the one million viewers in January 2004 would think differently. The TV producer for my documentary treated me with the utmost respect, so I felt my story was worth telling the viewers. The female producer kept me informed at every stage in the production of the documentary, and she didn't make cheap comments at my expense before, during, or after filming. She's an absolute sweetie, she really is.

Regrettably, a certain Lawrence Barraclough couldn't be trusted, and there's a good chance he took me for a sap. Some incidents are still worth repeating, and his documentary, first shown on BBC3, did not accurately represent what I had said in front of the cameras. An hour and a half interview in my house was whittled down to a two-minute segment, while my main statements were completely left out. Mr Barraclough's comments about me were inaccurate, and his statement that the penoplasty procedure was uncommon in this country is a downright lie. In fact the procedure is very popular in the United Kingdom—that's a statement of fact. I will put on the record again that he promised Sally Morgan he would let her do an interview with him. That was totally overlooked, and he never even had the decency to apologise to Sally. What a rat!

The other thing I should add is that his programmes are now seen on many free-to-air channels—so they can be repeated for the thousandth time. I'll never forget his statement to his viewing public, 'I discovered my problem was in my head and not my pants.' When I was channel-hopping earlier this year, what did I see, none other than Mr Barraclough with his first programme, *My Penis and I*. If you ask me, I

'A Little Bit of What You Fancy Does You Good'

think he has a problem in his head and his pants. He asks women their opinion on penis size and when they say that small ones do not turn them on, he totally ignores their replies. He doesn't realise that a little bit of what you fancy does us a heap of good, although the phrase 'a little bit' doesn't mean a woman has to put up with a tiny penis just to protect the ego of the bloke. That said, it also doesn't mean she has to say, 'How are you going to satisfy me with that tiny thing you pathetic little man?' There are ways of letting a gentleman down gently.

I couldn't sit through his bloody programme again, so I switched over to see another programme (I think it was a programme about the Second World War)—anything's better than his view of the world, where only men with tiny penises will inherit the earth. To Mr Barraclough I would simply say, 'Never mind the micropenises, here's the truth.'

CHAPTER SEVENTEEN

'Gigantic'

And this I know
His teeth as white as snow
What a gas it was to see him
Walk her every day
Into a shady place
With her lips, she said
She said

Hey Paul, Hey Paul, Hey Paul, let's have a ball [3x]

Gigantic, gigantic, gigantic
A big, big, love
Gigantic, gigantic, gigantic
A big, big, love

Lovely legs they are
What a big black mess
What a hunk of love
Walk her every day into a shady place
He's like the dark, but I'd want him

'Gigantic'

Hey Paul, Hey Paul, Hey Paul, let's have a ball [3x]

Gigantic, gigantic, gigantic
A big, big, love
Gigantic, gigantic, gigantic
A big, big, love

What do these lyrics mean? How long is a piece of string? Or, more importantly, how long is a penis?

The song was written by the Pixies, an American alternative rock band, who have been extremely influential since they formed in 1986. Regarding the above song, many people have their own perception of what the song actually means.

On the Internet, someone posted the following, 'This was written and sung by Kim Deal, who said she took inspiration from a 1986 Bruce Beresford movie, *Crimes of the Heart*. In the film, Sissy Spacek plays a married woman who falls in love with a black teenager.'

Another post said, 'Apple used this song in their iPhone ad campaign *Powerful*, which demonstrates how the consumer has "the power to create, shape and share" his or her life when they acquire the device.'

On the Daily Caller website, it says the following, 'The song seems euphoric as the actors sing out, "Gigantic, gigantic, gigantic / A big, big, love". What they don't say is that "Gigantic" is all about a large black penis.'

Another individual posted this simple message, 'I find it hilarious that a phone commercial chose a song about a big black dick.'

I've used the above song to illustrate that well-endowed men can be sung about in rock songs as well as be mentioned in erotic literature and, of course, shown in porn movies. They can also be shown on 'serious' TV documentaries. On first hearing the song, I must admit that I thought there was a hidden meaning about a well-endowed black guy, although I did think my conclusions were a bit too obvious. However, other people have said it was an 'unambiguous' song about a black guy who had a very large penis.

I described in my first book how I watched a series of TV documentaries (or, as some people call them, cockumentaries) on channel four, about the male organ. In one programme, entitled *The Biggest Penis in the World*, one woman said that if you simply google bigcocks.com on your computer, you would actually see couples having sex where the male 'star' would be extremely well hung.

Regarding the three programmes that made up the documentaries shown by channel four they were described thus,

Episode One—'The Perfect Penis': 'For some men bigger—whether by mechanical, herbal, or surgical means—will always mean better. The penis is the organ most central to a man's sense of self, and the quest for penile perfection has driven some men to extraordinary and sometimes dangerous lengths.'

Episode Two—'Chopped Off: The Man Who Lost His Penis': 'In 1993 one short brutal act guaranteed John Wayne Bobbitt a notoriety he can never shake off.'

Episode Three—'The World's Biggest Penis': 'No doubt about it, society celebrates the big penis. Seen as a sign of adequacy, virility, and manliness, those lucky enough to be well endowed are heralded by both sexes and all sexualities.'

These programmes were aired in 2009, when I was fifty-six, so that when I saw episode three, in which a woman mentioned the website bigcocks.com, I felt like the oldest person who was viewing porn movies for the first time. It felt as though I was old enough to be a grandfather, yet at the same time, I had never seen any of this stuff now freely available via your computer.

As I mentioned in my first book, I must have been left open-mouthed watching on my computer as the couples were seen having sexual intercourse and performing various other sexual acts. It remains the only time I've witnessed this material (with the exception of the website I mentioned earlier, namely tinydicks.com).

Four different 'films', lasting approximately five minutes each, showed four different men, all magnificently endowed, with four physically beautiful women, who all had perfect figures and large breasts. All the men had their cocks measured by the respective women. One guy measured nine and a half inches in length when erect, and after this they made love, if that's the right phrase, until they both reached orgasm. The second guy measured in at just over ten inches in length, and his penis was extremely thick in girth. They made love until he withdrew his penis so his ejaculation could be filmed. The third guy measured ten and a half inches in length, and he too had a very thick penis. Their lovemaking was extremely passionate, and he too withdrew so his ejaculation was filmed, ands he shot his load onto the woman's breasts. The biggest was left to last, as he was given the name of 'Mr One-Foot-Long'. The woman sounded astounded as she measured his incredible penis, which did indeed reach the twelve-inch mark on a steel ruler. His girth was so thick that she could only get her hand halfway around the thickest part of his penis. She masturbated him until he ejaculated into a clear plastic beaker. What shocked her (and me!) was that he spurted out his semen nine times before subsiding. I remembered distinctly as the woman said, 'Look how much come you've produced.'

All the above is the absolute truth and nothing but the truth. I will never view another porn film under the banner bigcocks.com, for the simple reason that it would make me feel so inadequate all over again that it's simply not worth the pain of it. Since my operations, I've definitely felt better about myself, and it's not worth watching men that leave me feeling as though I'm worthless. I watched this particular material firstly for research purposes—for my book—and secondly out of curiosity.

MICROPENIS: The Long and Short of It

I will say, however, that the series on channel five—*A Girl's Guide To 21st Century Sex*—was in some ways just as explicit as the films shown on bigcocks.com. In fact, the clever photography used on the channel five programmes used tiny cameras inside the woman's vagina to show her reaching orgasm as well as the man's ejaculation inside her vagina. This was permissible, don't forget, because it was deemed to be 'educational'. The series can still be seen on the Internet, so now's your chance, if you missed the series when it was first shown here in the United Kingdom. It begs the question though, what is considered educational and what is considered pornography?

Other things that were shown on *A Girl's Guide to 21st Century Sex* included three guys having their erections measured on the show because they all wanted to be bigger. The guy who was originally six and a half inches long when erect ended up extending that to seven and a half inches long. Boy did he look happy! There was a young woman seen masturbating because she could actually 'ejaculate' vaginal fluid or 'love juice'. A man who cheated on his wife had part of his penis cut off, although surgery managed to attach it back on. The man who was seen actually having sexual intercourse with his partner was also seen 'rimming' her for their mutual pleasure.

I've an idea that if these things were shown on the Internet, and they were not claimed to be 'educational', they might well be classified as pornography.

Being measured on screen on terrestrial television so millions of people could see I still had a micropenis would make me feel absolutely worthless. I did appear on channel five's documentary *Drastic Plastic* when I was seen on camera fully naked so my penis and balls were there for all to see. After my girth enhancement surgery, Dr Horn did measure my penis on camera to show what increase l had been given. In a way I feel proud about it, but then again I still feel inadequate when I compare myself to Anthony, who already had eight inches when erect but wanted to be bigger.

'Gigantic'

As Anna Camilleri has pointed out in the front of this book, 'Penoplasty is popular in the porn industry where, as they say, they are paid by the inch.' Just think, if I was measured at my original size preop in 1996, I wouldn't even be paid the minimum wage!

Nevertheless, to be told by someone like RP, who is also mentioned earlier in this book, that he found the motivation to have the penoplasty operation after reading my first book, it makes me feel both humble and very proud that he took my book so seriously. Quite simply, he believed in my story—what a compliment to give me.

Good luck to everyone out there, and I hope you have found this book helpful.